AGE-RELATED
MACULAR DEGENERATION

Current Management

AGE-RELATED
MACULAR DEGENERATION

Current Management

Editors

Jay S. Duker, MD
Andre J. Witkin, MD

New England Eye Center
Tufts University School of Medicine
Boston, Massachusetts

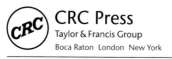

CRC Press
Taylor & Francis Group
Boca Raton London New York

CRC Press is an imprint of the
Taylor & Francis Group, an **informa** business

First published 2015 by SLACK Incorporated

Published 2024 by CRC Press
2385 NW Executive Center Drive, Suite 320, Boca Raton FL 33431

and by CRC Press
4 Park Square, Milton Park, Abingdon, Oxon, OX14 4RN

CRC Press is an imprint of Taylor & Francis Group, LLC

:

Library of Congress Cataloging in Publication Control Number: 2014018722

ISBN: 9781617116421 (pbk)
ISBN: 9781003522553 (ebk)

DOI: 10.1201/9781003522553

DEDICATION

I dedicate this book to my wife, Julie. Without her love, companionship, support, and respect, I would never be able to commit to the investment of time and effort a book like this represents.

—Jay S. Duker, MD

To my daughter Nora Bea, who will likely never read this book.

—Andre J. Witkin, MD

CONTENTS

ABOUT THE EDITORS

Jay S. Duker, MD is professor and chair of the Department of Ophthalmology at Tufts Medical Center and Tufts University School of Medicine and the Director of the New England Eye Center in Boston. Dr. Duker received his medical degree magna cum laude from Jefferson Medical College in Philadelphia. He completed an internal medicine internship at the Beth Israel Hospital in Boston. Dr. Duker then completed an ophthalmology residency, serving as chief resident, followed by a retina and vitreous surgery fellowship, at the Wills Eye Hospital in Philadelphia.

Dr. Duker's major research interests include imaging of the posterior segment, retinal vascular disease, and drug delivery to the posterior segment. He has pursued those interests as a coinvestigator or principal investigator of numerous studies funded by the National Institutes of Health/National Eye Institute, Massachusetts Institute of Technology, and industry, including studies of optical coherence tomography and several phase III trials. Specializing in medical and surgical diseases of the posterior segment, his surgical expertise includes macular diseases, retinal detachment, proliferative vitreoretinopathy, diabetic retinopathy, and intraocular tumors. He has published more than 180 journal articles, and he has been lead editor on 3 books and 13 book chapters. In addition, Dr. Duker lectures extensively both nationally and internationally. He is an associate editor of *Ophthalmic Surgery and Laser Therapy* and has served on the editorial boards of *Review of Ophthalmology*, *Evidence-Based Eye Care*, and *Retina Today*. He has been a reviewer for many journals, including *Ophthalmology*, *American Journal of Ophthalmology*, *Archives of Ophthalmology*, *Ophthalmic Surgery and Lasers*, *Retina*, and *The New England Journal of Medicine*, among others. Dr. Duker is the recipient of the Honor Award and Senior Honor Award from the American Academy of Ophthalmology.

Andre J. Witkin, MD was born in Waterville, Maine. He attended Dartmouth College, earning his bachelor's degree magna cum laude with high honors in biology. He earned his MD from Weill Cornell Medical College in New York City and did his ophthalmology residency at the New England Eye Center of Tufts Medical Center in Boston. Dr. Witkin then did a 2-year fellowship in retinal disease and vitreoretinal surgery at the Wills Eye Institute in Philadelphia. In 2012, he joined the ophthalmology faculty at the New England Eye Center of Tufts Medical Center as an assistant professor. Dr. Witkin has a special interest in clinical research, particularly in the field of retinal imaging. He has published more than 30 articles in peer-reviewed journals and several book chapters and has presented at more than a dozen national meetings in the field of ophthalmology. Dr. Witkin is currently the primary investigator for a number of clinical trials in macular degeneration and central serous chorioretinopathy at the New England Eye Center.

CONTRIBUTING AUTHORS

Anita Agarwal, MD (Chapter 1)
Professor of Ophthalmology
Retina, Vitreous, and Uveitis
Vanderbilt Eye Institute
Nashville, Tennessee

Sophie J. Bakri, MD (Chapter 5)
Professor of Ophthalmology
Mayo Clinic Department of Ophthalmology
Rochester, Minnesota

Christopher J. Brady, MD (Chapters 8, 9)
Retina Fellow
Wills Eye Hospital Retina Service
Philadelphia, Pennsylvania

Sunir J. Garg, MD, FACS (Chapter 4, Section 1)
Associate Professor of Ophthalmology
Mid Atlantic Retina
The Retina Service of Wills Eye Hospital
Thomas Jefferson University
Philadelphia, Pennsylvania

Roger A. Goldberg, MD, MBA (Chapter 10)
Ophthalmic Consultants of Boston
Tufts New England Eye Center
Boston, Massachusetts

Jeffrey S. Heier, MD (Chapter 10)
Ophthalmic Consultants of Boston
Boston, Massachusetts

S.K. Steven Houston III, MD (Chapter 4, Section 1)
Retina Fellow
Mid Atlantic Retina
The Retina Service of Wills Eye Hospital
Thomas Jefferson University
Philadelphia, Pennsylvania

Kapil G. Kapoor, MD (Chapter 5)
Assistant Professor of Ophthalmology
Eastern Virginia Medical School
Department of Ophthalmology
Wagner Macula & Retina Center
Virginia Beach, Virginia

Nora M.V. Laver, MD (Chapter 2)
Associate Professor of Ophthalmology and Pathology
Tufts University School of Medicine
Associate Clinical Professor of Oral and Maxillofacial Pathology
Tufts School of Dental Medicine
Boston, Massachusetts

Sana Nadeem, MBBS (Chapter 3)
Senior Registrar
Fauji Foundation Hospital
Rawalpindi, Pakistan

Llewelyn J. Rao, MD (Chapter 7)
Retina Associates of Cleveland
Cleveland, Ohio

Carl D. Regillo, MD (Chapter 9)
Director, Retina Service
Wills Eye Hospital
Professor of Ophthalmology
Thomas Jefferson University
Philadelphia, Pennsylvania

Elias Reichel, MD (Chapter 4, Section 3)
Professor of Ophthalmology
Director of the Vitreoretinal Diseases and Surgery Service
Department of Ophthalmology
Tufts Medical Center
Boston, Massachusetts

Philip J. Rosenfeld, MD, PhD (Chapter 6)
Bascom Palmer Eye Institute
University of Miami
Miller School of Medicine
Miami, Florida

Chirag P. Shah, MD, MPH (Chapter 8)
Ophthalmic Consultants of Boston
Boston, Massachusetts

Lawrence J. Singerman, MD, FACS (Chapter 7)
Retina Associates of Cleveland
Cleveland, Ohio

Mariana R. Thorell, MD (Chapter 6)
Bascom Palmer Eye Institute
University of Miami
Miller School of Medicine
Miami, Florida

Michael D. Tibbetts, MD (Chapter 4, Section 3)
Cape Coral Eye Center
Cape Coral, Florida

Nadia K. Waheed, MD, MPH (Chapter 3)
Assistant Professor Ophthalmology
Tufts University Medical School and the New England Eye Center
Boston, Massachusetts

PREFACE

With advances in medicine that have helped to prolong life, the population of elderly individuals is expanding at an ever-increasing rate. Due to this trend, eye diseases that affect this age group, including cataract, glaucoma, and age-related macular degeneration (AMD), are becoming increasingly prevalent. Treatments for all of these conditions have advanced, but many people continue to lose central vision from AMD, which has become the leading cause of significant vision loss in developed countries in people older than age 65. For this reason, it is important for all eye care providers to be familiar with the most up-to-date aspects of the clinical management of AMD. This book is intended to summarize the most current clinically relevant aspects of the management of this potentially devastating disease and serve as a handbook and clinical reference for medical students, residents, fellows, general ophthalmologists, and retina specialists.

In the first chapter of this book, some of the key risk factors for the development of AMD are summarized. Although much is known regarding genetics and modifiable risk factors that affect the risk of developing AMD, it remains a mystery why some people develop the disease and others do not and why there is so much variability in disease phenotypes. In Chapters 2 and 3, the disease is classified based on both clinical and histopathological appearance, and aspects of pathology and clinical examination give further insight into the pathophysiology of the disease. Certain clinical characteristics on clinical examination have also been correlated with risk stratification for the development of more advanced forms of AMD, and these are summarized in Chapter 3.

The variety of imaging studies used to diagnose AMD are summarized in Chapter 4, and Chapter 5 describes some other macular diseases that may masquerade as AMD, which can be differentiated from AMD based on appearance and history and with retinal imaging. Fluorescein angiography and fundus photography are crucial to the diagnosis and management of AMD. Fundus autofluorescence and indocyanine green angiography have also become useful in diagnosis and management. More recently, optical coherence tomography has played a pivotal role in the diagnosis and management of AMD, particularly in the era of intravitreal injections for neovascular (wet) AMD.

Although the Age-Related Eye Disease Study (AREDS) found that certain vitamins may slow the progression of non-neovascular (dry) AMD, wet AMD is the subtype that most current treatment options are able to target. Chapters 6 through 9 discuss the key aspects of the management of wet AMD. In the past, focal laser photocoagulation was used as a primary treatment, and in the early 2000s this was supplanted by photodynamic therapy. These treatments slowed the progression of vision loss; however, patients still lost a significant amount of vision despite treatment. More recently, management of wet AMD was revolutionized with the introduction of intravitreal anti-vascular endothelial growth factor (anti-VEGF) medications, which were not only safe but able to halt vision loss in the vast majority of patients with wet AMD and improve visual acuity in a large number of patients.

Despite improvement in vision and macular anatomy in the majority of patients with wet AMD treated with anti-VEGF injections, a minority of these patients do not respond as well to treatment, and alternative clinical treatment approaches have been considered. When patients present with a large submacular hemorrhage, which does not typically respond as well to intravitreal injections, vitrectomy surgery may be attempted to salvage the central vision.

Finally, some future directions of AMD research are summarized in Chapter 10. Notably, much research is being done in the field of preventative treatments for patients with dry AMD, which is a subset of patients for whom we do not currently have good treatment options. Interestingly, many of the targets of current treatment research are also listed as genetic risk markers in Chapter 1.

We hope this book proves to be a handy reference for the wide variety of eye care professionals involved in the diagnosis and clinical management of AMD. We'd like to wholeheartedly thank the generous experts in the field that contributed to the writing of this book, as well as the editors at SLACK Incorporated who made this book possible.

Jay S. Duker, MD
Andre J. Witkin, MD

1

EPIDEMIOLOGY, GENETICS, AND MODIFIABLE RISK FACTORS

Anita Agarwal, MD

Age-related macular degeneration (AMD) is a prime example of a complex inherited disorder where genes, environment, and the individual interact in variable ways to manifest the disease. This chapter will discuss the epidemiology of AMD and the different known genetic and environmental risk factors associated with the disease.

EPIDEMIOLOGY OF AGE-RELATED MACULAR DEGENERATION

Globally, AMD ranks third among the causes of blindness, following cataract and glaucoma. However, it is the primary cause of blindness in industrialized nations. The estimated number of visually impaired individuals in the world is 285 million; 39 million are blind and 246 million have low vision. Sixty-five percent of all visually impaired and 82% of all blind individuals are aged 50 years and older. In 2004, approximately 21 million older adults were affected by AMD worldwide.[1]

Estimates of the prevalence of AMD are mostly based on cumulative data from major epidemiological studies: the Beaver Dam Eye Study (BDES),[2] Blue Mountains Eye Study,[3] National Health and Nutrition Examination Survey,[4] Barbados Eye Study (BES),[5] Rotterdam Study,[6] Framingham Eye Study,[7,8] Chesapeake Bay Waterman Study,[9] and Baltimore Eye Survey.[10] The prevalence of AMD in these groups varies based on their definition of AMD. The BDES revealed a population prevalence of 1.8% of advanced stages of AMD, of which 1.2% had neovascular (wet) AMD in at least one eye and 0.6% had geographic atrophy secondary to non-neovascular (dry) AMD.[2] The prevalence of advanced stages of AMD increased with age to 7.1% in individuals aged 75 years and older.

The Framingham Eye Study used age-specific, 5-year prevalence data to estimate incidence rates.[8] The incidence rates were 2.5%, 6.7%, and 10.8% for individuals aged 65, 70, and 75 years, respectively. The incidence of early AMD rose from 3.9% in individuals aged 43 to 54 years to 22.8% for those aged 75 years and older. The BES described a 4-year incidence of 5.2% for early AMD.[5] The incidence of advanced AMD was low in this group.

Duker JS, Witkin AJ, eds.
Age-Related Macular Degeneration:
Current Management (pp. 1-14)
© 2015 Taylor & Francis Group

More recently, prediction models have been created to forecast the risk of advanced AMD in a given population. Age, sex, and genetic and environmental risk factors (discussed later) were considered in the prediction model. The 3-continent consortium consisted of the Rotterdam Study, the BDES, and the Blue Mountains Eye Study.[11] Their model included age, sex, 26 single-nucleotide polymorphisms in AMD risk genes, smoking, body mass index, and baseline AMD phenotype. Individuals with low-risk scores had a hazard ratio of 0.02 (95% confidence interval [CI]) to develop advanced AMD, whereas individuals with high-risk scores had a hazard ratio of 22.0 (95% CI). Cumulative risk of advanced AMD incidence ranged from nearly 0 to more than 65% for those with the highest risk scores.[11]

Evidence exists that a variant of wet AMD, termed *polypoidal choroidal vasculopathy*, is more prevalent in Asian populations compared with White populations. Polypoidal choroidal vasculopathy may account for up to 50% of cases of wet AMD in Asian populations and only 8% to 13% of wet AMD cases in White populations.[12] This is an important distinction because there may be different genetic markers associated with this AMD variant, and it may respond differently to treatment, as discussed in later chapters.

PATHOLOGY AND PATHOPHYSIOLOGY OF AGE-RELATED MACULAR DEGENERATION

The pathology of AMD is discussed in more detail in Chapter 2, but some key aspects of the pathology and pathophysiology of AMD are briefly summarized in this chapter to aid in the discussion of known genetic polymorphisms and their relationship to the development of AMD. Drusen are one of the first visible signs of AMD and form the basis of definition and diagnosis of early AMD. Drusen are deposits of extracellular material that accumulate under the retinal pigment epithelium (RPE) between the basement membrane of the RPE and Bruch's membrane. Drusen are composed of extracellular membrane proteins such as vitronectin,[13-15] clusterin (apolipoprotein E),[16,17] complement activators and components of the complement cascade,[14] amyloid p,[18] lipofuscin constituents (eg, A2E),[19,20] C-reactive protein,[21] cholesterol,[22,23] immunoglobulins,[24] immune complexes,[25,26] and advanced glycation end products.[27]

Age-related changes in the RPE/Bruch's membrane complex resemble atherosclerotic changes occurring in blood vessel walls, with accumulation of unesterified cholesterol. In addition, thickening of Bruch's membrane occurs, likely mediated in part by impaired interaction of matrix metalloproteinases and tissue inhibitors of metalloproteinases (TIMPs).[28] Lipid-rich basal laminar and basal linear deposits accumulate in Bruch's membrane. The RPE cells accumulate lipofuscin and A2E, which are byproducts of photoreceptor turnover. Over time, the overlying photoreceptors lose cell bodies and die. When the interaction between the photoreceptors and RPE is lost due to death of photoreceptors, the RPE migrate and die, resulting in geographic atrophy. Late changes in AMD also show evidence of angiogenesis, mediated by production of vascular endothelial growth factor (VEGF).

Thus, inflammation and immune processes signified by the presence of complement activators and immunoglobulins, alterations in collagen and extracellular matrix (ECM) proteins, lipid accumulation, cell death, and angiogenesis are all participants in the pathogenesis of AMD. Genes involved in many of these pathways have been found to be associated with AMD (Table 1-1).

TABLE 1-1. GENES ASSOCIATED WITH
AGE-RELATED MACULAR DEGENERATION

GENE	PROTEIN	CHROMOSOME
Complement		
CFH	Complement factor H	1q32
CFHR 1-5	CFH-related proteins 1-5	1q32
CF3	Complement factor 3	6p21
C2	Complement component 2	6p21
CFI	Complement factor I	4q25
C3	Complement component 3	19p13
CFD	Complement factor D	19p13
CFB	Complement factor B (properdin)	6p21
SERPING1	Complement 1 inhibitor protein	11q12
Immunity (Other Than Complement)		
RORA	Retinoic acid receptor–related orphan receptor α	15q21
CX3CR1	Fractalkine receptor	3p21
HLA-C	Human leukocyte antigen C	6p21
IL8	Interleukin 8	4q13
TL4	Toll-like receptor 4	9q33
F13B	β-subunit of coagulation factor XIII	1q31
PLEKHA1	Tandem pleckstrin-homology domain-containing protein 1	10q26
TNFRSF10A	Tumor necrosis factor receptor super-family 10a	8p21
Extracellular Matrix		
HTRA1	High temperature requirement A protein	10q26
ARMS2	Age-related maculopathy susceptibility protein 2	10q26
FBLN6/ HMCN1	Fibulin-6	1q25
ROBO1	Roundabout homolog 1	3p12
CST3	Cystatin 3	20p11
COL8A1	Collagen type 8 α1 subunit	3q12

(continued)

TABLE 1-1 (CONTINUED). GENES ASSOCIATED WITH AGE-RELATED MACULAR DEGENERATION

GENE	PROTEIN	CHROMOSOME
Extracellular Matrix		
COL10A1	Fyn-related kinase/α-chain of type X collagen	6q21
TIMP3	Tissue inhibitor of metalloproteinase 3	22q12
Lipid Transportation		
ABCA1	ATP-binding cassette protein 1	9q31
ABCA4	ATP-binding cassette protein 4	1p22
ApoE	Apolipoprotein E	19q13
CETP	Cholesterol ester transfer protein	16q21
CYP24A1	Cytochrome p450 family	20q13
ELOVL4	ELOVL fatty acid elongase 4	6q14
FADS1-3	Fatty acid desaturase 1-3	11q12
LIPC/LPL	Hepatic lipase/lipoprotein lipase	15q21
VLDLR	Very light density lipoprotein receptor	9p24
Angiogenesis		
SERPINF1	Pigment epithelium-derived factor	17p13
VEGFA	Vascular endothelial growth factor A	6p12

GENETICS OF AGE-RELATED MACULAR DEGENERATION

The genetics of AMD is extremely complex and has been a topic of extensive research. Early gene studies found only modest association (5% to 7%) of the genes APOE, ABCA4, and fibulin-5 with AMD.[29-31] With rapid improvements in gene extraction technologies, the first major breakthrough occurred in 2005 with the simultaneous discovery by 4 different groups of polymorphisms in the complement factor H (CFH) gene in patients with AMD.[32-35] Subsequent to this, the second major set of AMD genes, HTRA1/ARMS2, was found on chromosome 10.[36] Since then, 2 major loci, 1q32 and 10q26, have been identified as regions of the most significant interest in association with AMD.[37] The 1q32 locus contains genes involved in inflammation and immune function, collectively called the regulators of complement activation gene cluster, which is made up of the CFH and CFH-related (CFHR1-5) genes. The 10q26 region has the HTRA1/ARMS2 genes that encode a number of the high-temperature requirement family of proteases. More recently, other pathogenetic genes have been sought by combining data from several large groups from around the world (ie, AMD Gene Consortium) and by using genome-wide association studies.[38] This has yielded several loci, such as TIMP3, high-density lipoprotein, and others.[39] Some genes associated with AMD and their possible role in the pathogenesis of this disease are discussed in the sections that follow.

Complement System and Immunity

Mutations in CFH (1q32), resulting in an increased risk of AMD, were first reported in 2005, and CFH represented the first gene identified that had a significant association with AMD. Strong associations between the Y402H polymorphism in the CFH gene and AMD susceptibility were found with a population-attributable risk of 25% to 50%.[32-35] A highly-penetrant mutation (H5) confers an even higher risk of AMD, with a more severe and earlier onset of the disease. Five genes within the regulators of complement activation gene cluster encode CFH-related proteins (CFHR1-5).[40,41] They lack the N-terminal complement regulatory region but have the C-terminal surface binding regions. CFHR3, 4, and 5 each bind C3b and are believed to enhance CFH-mediated C3b degradation. The effects of CFHR polymorphisms on AMD risk depend on the complex interactions among the CFHR and CFH genes. Some polymorphisms are protective, such as a common deletion of CFHR1 and CFHR3, whereas others are associated with a higher risk of AMD, such as a rare deletion of CFHR1 and CFHR4 associated with bilateral geographic atrophy.

Complement factor B (CFB) and complement component 2 (C2)[42-44] on 6p21.3, and 2 nonsynonymous polymorphisms in the C3/CFD (19p13.3-p13.2) gene, have also been reported to be associated with AMD.[45,46] They are involved in the classic, lectin, and alternate pathways of complement activation. Polymorphisms in CFI on 4q25 seem to be associated with advanced AMD.[47,48] F13B (1q31-q32.1) encodes the β-subunit of coagulation factor XIII, which regulates platelet adhesion and fibrin cross-linking, thus stabilizing fibrin clots and ECM.[49]

The interaction of CFH, CFB, and the C3 triad appears to be a defining feature of AMD genetic susceptibility. Combined analyses of the CFH and CFB/C2 variants have been shown to account for nearly 75% of all AMD cases in the European and North American populations.[40] Complement dysregulation leading to inflammation appears to be the major factor in the pathogenesis of AMD. Multiple complement proteins are found in drusen, RPE, Bruch's membrane, basal laminar deposits, retina, and the choriocapillaris. In particular, the CFH Y402 variant and PLEKHA1 are major participants in complement pathway dysregulation.[50]

SERPING1 on 11q12-q13.1 encodes complement 1 inhibitor protein, which regulates complement activation by inhibiting activated C1r and C1s. Deficiency in the C1 inhibitor results in production of excess bradykinin, which increases vascular permeability and inflammation.[51] Polymorphisms in SERPING1 have been associated with AMD.

The RORA gene encodes retinoic acid receptor–related orphan receptor α. Polymorphisms of this gene itself and in association with polymorphisms in HTRA1/ARMS2 are known to increase the risk of AMD. The CX3CR1 gene product is a receptor for fractalkine, a transmembrane protein and chemokine that regulates leukocyte adhesion and cell migration.[52-54] Polymorphisms in this gene may interfere with inflammatory cell recruitment, which is necessary to clear debris and deposits, thus increasing the risk of AMD. Other polymorphisms in the human leukocyte antigen HLA-C, IL8, and the toll-like receptors TL3 and TL4 have also been associated with AMD[55-57]; TL3 decreases risk, whereas the rest increase risk of AMD.

Extracellular Matrix, Collagen, and Cell Adhesion

The second major risk locus, 10q26, contains 3 genes—PLEKHA1, ARMS2, and HTRA1.[50] Their functions have not been fully elucidated, but they are thought to be involved in immunity, cellular homeostasis, and ECM integrity. PLEKHA1 (10q26.13) encodes TAPP1, which regulates B-cell activation and antibody production, again implying an immunologic basis of the pathogenesis of AMD. ARMS2 is found in several tissues, including the intercapillary pillars of the choroid. It codes for a protein of undetermined function that binds to the ECM proteins fibronectin-1, fibulin-6, and elastin microfibril. ARMS2 has also been shown to localize to mitochondria.[58] Oxidative stress may alter mitochondrial function, thus affecting cell survival. High temperature requirement A (HTRA1) (10q26.3) encodes one of the HTRA family of proteases, which are heat shock proteins that cleave misfolded or denatured proteins and are therefore necessary for cell survival. The HTRA1 protein also demonstrates elastase activity, which may contribute to changes in Bruch's membrane. It may also regulate insulin-like growth factor II, which is known to promote angiogenesis, thus potentially playing a role in development of neovascular AMD.

The association of F13B (1q32) and ARMS2/HTRA1 (10q26) with AMD signifies the role of the ECM in AMD pathogenesis.[49] Pathologic changes in Bruch's membrane, which is composed of elastin and collagen, occur at many stages of AMD and may be affected by polymorphisms in genes that regulate ECM structure and function.

Fibulin-5 (FBLN5; 14q32.1) promotes elastic fiber assembly and maturation and is found in Bruch's membrane and the choriocapillaris in normal eyes. In AMD eyes, it has been found in sub-RPE deposits and drusen. It may interact with HTRA1 to disrupt ECM integrity.[31] Fibulin-6 (FBLN6; HMCN1) is structurally similar to the protein produced by EFEMP1, one of the genes associated with autosomal-dominant forms of macular degeneration (Malattia leventinese or Doyne's honeycomb retinal dystrophy). Other genes involved in ECM alteration include ROBO1, CST3, COL8A1, COL10A1, and TIMP3.[39,59-65]

Lipid Transportation and Metabolism

Lipid accumulation in drusen and basal linear deposits are major factors in AMD pathology. Several genes involved in lipid metabolism and transport have been implicated in AMD.

ABCA1 encodes a cholesterol efflux pump in the cellular lipid removal pathway, and ABCA4 encodes retina-specific adenosine triphosphate (ATP)-binding cassette protein (ABCR), which functions in clearing all-*trans*-retinal. Abnormalities of the ABCR protein lead to accumulation of A2E and lipofuscin in the RPE. The ABCA4 gene is mutated in autosomal-recessive Stargardt's disease and has been associated with AMD in some studies.[66,67] The ApoE (19q13.2) gene, a major component of drusen, is involved in catabolism of triglyceride-rich lipoproteins in the liver, thus maintaining normal lipid homeostasis. The E4 haplotype of ApoE is associated with decreased risk of AMD, whereas individuals with the E2/E2 homozygous haplotypes carry a higher risk of AMD.[29] ApoE is also synthesized in response to neuronal injury and stress, hence fragments of ApoE may be neurotoxic.

Cholesterol ester transfer protein (CETP) is localized to the inter-photoreceptor matrix and may be part of the internal lipid transport system of the retina. The Genome-Wide Association Study reported an association with CETP in advanced AMD.[39] CYP24A1 is a member of the cytochrome p450 family of enzymes and is involved in the degradation of D3, a cholesterol derivative. Several mutations in this gene have been associated with increased AMD risk.[65] Other genes involved in lipid metabolism and transport include ELOVL4, which encodes ELOVL fatty acid elongase, a protein that has been associated with Stargardt-like macular dystrophy, as well as AMD.[50] FADS1-3, LIPCLPL, and LRP6 are other lipid-associated genes that are thought to be associated with AMD.

Angiogenesis

Angiogenesis is a normal response of tissue to injury and inflammation. However, genetic susceptibility to early or more severe angiogenesis may play a role in the development of neovascular AMD.

The SERPINF1 (17p13.3) gene codes pigment epithelium-derived factor, which is a potent inhibitor of angiogenesis. Mutations in the SERPINF1 gene may affect this inhibition, thus increasing risk for wet AMD.[68] VEGFA (6p12) encodes VEGF. Polymorphisms in the VEGFA gene have been associated with a higher risk of neovascular AMD. VEGFA is known to play a key role in the development and progression of neovascular AMD because inhibitors of this molecule have now become the mainstay for treatment of this disease (see Chapter 6). VLDLR (9p24) modulates angiogenesis and plays a role in neovascular AMD pathogenesis. Another gene involved in angiogenesis is HTRA1, which acts by its interaction with ECM and other regulatory proteins (see previous section).

GENETIC TESTING

Recently, genetic testing has become commercially available to clinicians and patients. Currently, 2 companies make genetic testing kits that may be used in the clinic: Macula Risk PGx (ArcticDx, Inc) and RetinaGene AMD (Nicox). These kits test for specific AMD-related, single-nucleotide polymorphisms in some of the genes listed in this chapter, which have been linked to AMD. Both tests are intended to be used in patients with dry AMD, and both tests give a 2-, 5- and 10-year risk score of progression to advanced AMD. Currently, it remains unclear as to what role these genetic tests play in the clinic, and the American Academy of Ophthalmology does not recommend the routine use of these tests.[69] However, in the future, this type of genetic testing may accurately assess risk of AMD progression and may direct targeted therapies for patients with specific genetic polymorphisms.

MODIFIABLE RISK FACTORS OF AGE-RELATED MACULAR DEGENERATION

Aging is the strongest risk factor for AMD, but, of course, it is not modifiable. Age-related changes in Bruch's membrane and age-related formation of the components of drusen, as described earlier, play the strongest role in AMD.[70] Other risk factors that are modifiable have also been implicated in the development and/or progression of AMD and are discussed in the sections that follow.

Smoking

Smoking is the most significant and consistent modifiable risk factor associated with AMD and has been verified in many studies.[71,72] A history of smoking increases the susceptibility of genetically prone individuals to the development of advanced forms of AMD, sometimes even doubling the incidence.[70,73,74] Nicotine and other products in smoke have been found to increase the size of choroidal new vessels and the vascular smooth muscles in experimental animals,[75] alter the RPE membrane, and increase formation of sub-RPE deposits.[76]

Vitamins

One of the most well-known AMD trials was the Age-Related Eye Disease Study (AREDS), which demonstrated that daily oral supplementation with high doses of antioxidant vitamins and minerals in patients with intermediate dry AMD in both eyes or advanced AMD in the fellow eye reduced the risk of developing advanced AMD by 25% at 5 years (see Chapter 3).[77] The standard AREDS formulation consists of the following:

- β-carotene (vitamin A): 15 mg
- Vitamin C: 500 mg
- Vitamin E: 400 IU
- Zinc oxide: 80 mg
- Cupric oxide: 2 mg

Of note, β-carotene has since been associated with a small increased risk of lung cancer in current or former tobacco smokers, and patients who are current or former smokers should be advised to take the AREDS-based supplement with lutein/zeaxantin in place of β-carotene.

The antioxidant carotenoids lutein and zeaxanthin are found in dark green or yellow vegetables and are present in high concentrations in the macula. The exact protective role of these macular pigments remains uncertain; it has been proposed that their antioxidant effects may limit the damaging photo-oxidative effects of blue light. Studies have shown that increased intake of lutein and zeaxanthin and foods rich in these nutrients (eg, spinach and kale) are associated with a decreased risk of wet AMD.[78] Dietary analyses of the observational component of the AREDS also showed that lutein and zeaxanthin reduced the risk of AMD progression.[79]

The AREDS2 more recently evaluated a modification of the AREDS formula without β-carotene, with a lower dose of zinc (25 mg), and with the addition of 10 mg of lutein and 2 mg of zeaxanthin (as well as adding omega-3 fatty acids; discussed later in this chapter).[80] Replacement of the standard dose of zinc (80 mg) with the lower dose of zinc and the replacement of β-carotene with lutein/zeaxanthin did not decrease the effectiveness of the AREDS formulation in reducing the risk of AMD progression. However, the AREDS2 showed no increased benefit of adding of supplemental dietary lutein/zeaxanthin to the standard AREDS formulation.[80] Therefore, it is unclear whether the addition of lutein/zeaxanthin provides additional benefit to the original AREDS formulation.

Vitamin D has also been implicated in AMD. In studies of identical twins, the twin with a lower dietary vitamin D intake was found to have more severe AMD compared with the twin who had a higher intake.[81] Serum 25-hydroxyvitamin D was also found to be lower in patients with more severe AMD.[82]

Omega-3 Fatty Acids

Omega-3 fatty acids are found in photoreceptor outer segments. The primary dietary omega-3 fatty acids that have been studied in AMD are docosahexaenoic acid (DHA) and eicosapentaenoic acid (EPA), which are mostly found in fatty fishes such as salmon and sardines. DHA is a structural component of the retina, whereas EPA may play a role in retinal function and signaling.[80] Other dietary sources of omega-3 fatty acids, such as walnuts and flax seeds, primarily contain α-linolenic acid, which the body then converts to DHA and EPA. Observational studies have supported the beneficial effects of omega-3 fatty acids on AMD.[79,83,84] However, the AREDS2 recently showed that the addition of DHA (350 mg) and EPA (650 mg) to the AREDS formula did not further decrease the risk of progression to advanced AMD,[80] and it remains unclear whether the addition of an omega-3 fatty acid supplement to the AREDS formulation produces any additional benefit.

Fat-Rich Diet and Body Mass Index

A fat-rich diet has been associated with higher AMD risk, possibly by contributing to the lipid deposition on Bruch's membrane.[85-93] However, not all studies consistently show a link between fat intake and AMD risk. Many studies have implicated a higher body mass index to association with AMD; however, not all studies reveal a consistent association.[11,74,94-99] Individuals with AMD are also known to be at increased risk of cardiovascular disease and stroke.[100]

Sunlight

Sunlight has been shown to be associated with a higher incidence of AMD in some studies, but not in others. A recent meta-analysis of 14 studies has revealed a small, but significantly increased, risk of AMD with more sunlight exposure. This may be due to increased oxidative stress or direct-aging changes caused by increased photoreceptor/RPE activity.[101]

Other Risk Factors

Some studies have suggested that women may be associated with a higher risk of developing AMD.[102] Nonmodifiable ocular risk factors for AMD may include darker iris pigmentation,[103] previous cataract surgery,[104] and hyperopic refraction.[105] Some studies have suggested that previous cataract surgery is a risk factor for AMD,[102] but a secondary analysis of data from the AREDS showed no such association,[106] and it remains unclear whether cataract surgery is directly associated with a risk of AMD or AMD progression.

SUMMARY

AMD is an example of a complex inherited disorder resulting from variable interactions among genes, environment, and the individual. Research has made significant strides toward understanding the basis of this complex disorder. Work is ongoing toward finding ways to prevent or slow the progression of the condition.

REFERENCES

1. Mariotti SP, Pascolini D. Global estimates of visual impairment: 2010. *Br J Ophthalmol.* 2012;96(5):614-618.

2. Klein R, Lee KE, Gangnon RE, Klein BE. Incidence of visual impairment over a 20-year period: the Beaver Dam Eye Study. *Ophthalmology.* 2013;120:1210-1219.

3. Wang JJ, Rochtchina E, Lee AJ, et al. Ten-year incidence and progression of age-related maculopathy: the Blue Mountains Eye Study. *Ophthalmology.* 2007;114(1):92-98.

4. Weiner DE, Tighiouart H, Reynolds R, Seddon JM. Kidney function, albuminuria and age-related macular degeneration in NHANES III. *Nephrol Dial Transplant.* 2011;26:3159-3165.

5. Leske MC, Wu SY, Hennis A, et al. Nine-year incidence of age-related macular degeneration in the Barbados Eye Studies. *Ophthalmology.* 2006;113:29-35.

6. Vingerling JR, Hofman A, Grobbee DE, de Jong PT. Age-related macular degeneration and smoking. The Rotterdam Study. *Arch Ophthalmol.* 1996;114:1193-1196.

7. Rosenthal AR. The Framingham Eye Study: an editorial. *Surv Ophthalmol.* 1980;24:611-613.

8. Kahn HA, Leibowitz HM, Ganley JP, et al. The Framingham Eye Study. II. Association of ophthalmic pathology with single variables previously measured in the Framingham Heart Study. *Am J Epidemiol.* 1977;106:33-41.

9. Tikellis G, Robman LD, Harper CA, et al. The VECAT study: methodology and statistical power for measurement of age-related macular features. Vitamin E, Cataract, and Age-related Maculopathy Study. *Ophthalmic Epidemiol.* 1999;6(3):181-94

10. Rahmani B, Tielsch JM, Katz J, et al. The cause-specific prevalence of visual impairment in an urban population: the Baltimore Eye Survey. *Ophthalmology.* 1996;103(11):1721-1726.

11. Buitendijk GH, Rochtchina E, Myers C, et al. Prediction of age-related macular degeneration in the general population: the Three Continent AMD Consortium. *Ophthalmology.* 2013;120:2644-2655.

12. Laude A, Cackett PD, Vithana EN, et al. Polypoidal choroidal vasculopathy and neovascular age-related macular degeneration: same or different disease? *Prog Retin Eye Res.* 2010;29:19-29.

13. Anderson DH, Hageman GS, Mullins RF, et al. Vitronectin gene expression in the adult human retina. *Invest Ophthalmol Vis Sci.* 1999;40:3305-3315.

14. Hageman GS, Mullins RF. Molecular composition of drusen as related to substructural phenotype. *Mol Vis.* 1999;5:28.

15. Hageman GS, Mullins RF, Russell SR, Johnson LV, Anderson DH. Vitronectin is a constituent of ocular drusen and the vitronectin gene is expressed in human retinal pigmented epithelial cells. *FASEB J.* 1999;13:477-484.

16. Sakaguchi H, Miyagi M, Shadrach KG, Rayborn ME, Crabb JW, Hollyfield JG. Clusterin is present in drusen in age-related macular degeneration. *Exp Eye Res.* 2002;74:547-549.

17. Johnson LV, Leitner WP, Staples MK, Anderson DH. Complement activation and inflammatory processes in Drusen formation and age related macular degeneration. *Exp Eye Res.* 2001;73:887-896.

18. Anderson DH, Talaga KC, Rivest AJ, Barron E, Hageman GS, Johnson LV. Characterization of beta amyloid assemblies in drusen: the deposits associated with aging and age-related macular degeneration. *Exp Eye Res.* 2004;78:243-256.

19. Zhou J, Jang YP, Kim SR, Sparrow JR. Complement activation by photooxidation products of A2E, a lipofuscin constituent of the retinal pigment epithelium. *Proc Natl Acad Sci U S A.* 2006;103:16182-16187.

20. Zhou J, Kim SR, Westlund BS, Sparrow JR. Complement activation by bisretinoid constituents of RPE lipofuscin. *Invest Ophthalmol Vis Sci.* 2009;50:1392-1399.

21. Johnson PT, Betts KE, Radeke MJ, Hageman GS, Anderson DH, Johnson LV. Individuals homozygous for the age-related macular degeneration risk-conferring variant of complement factor H have elevated levels of CRP in the choroid. *Proc Natl Acad Sci U S A.* 2006;103:17456-17461.

22. Curcio CA, Millican CL, Bailey T, Kruth HS. Accumulation of cholesterol with age in human Bruch's membrane. *Invest Ophthalmol Vis Sci.* 2001;42:265-274.

23. Haimovici R, Gantz DL, Rumelt S, Freddo TF, Small DM. The lipid composition of drusen, Bruch's membrane, and sclera by hot stage polarizing light microscopy. *Invest Ophthalmol Vis Sci.* 2001;42:1592-1599.

24. Li CM, Chung BH, Presley JB, et al. Lipoprotein-like particles and cholesteryl esters in human Bruch's membrane: initial characterization. *Invest Ophthalmol Vis Sci.* 2005;46:2576-2586.

25. Johnson LV, Ozaki S, Staples MK, Erickson PA, Anderson DH. A potential role for immune complex pathogenesis in drusen formation. *Exp Eye Res.* 2000;70:441-449.

26. Mullins RF, Russell SR, Anderson DH, Hageman GS. Drusen associated with aging and age-related macular degeneration contain proteins common to extracellular deposits associated with atherosclerosis, elastosis, amyloidosis, and dense deposit disease. *FASEB J.* 2000;14:835-846.

27. Glenn JV, Mahaffy H, Wu K, et al. Advanced glycation end product (AGE) accumulation on Bruch's membrane: links to age-related RPE dysfunction. *Invest Ophthalmol Vis Sci.* 2009;50:441-451.

28. Hussain AA, Lee Y, Zhang JJ, Marshall J. Disturbed matrix metalloproteinase activity of Bruch's membrane in age-related macular degeneration. *IOVS.* 2011;52(7):4459-4466.

29. Schmidt S, Klaver C, Saunders A, et al. A pooled case-control study of the apolipoprotein E (APOE) gene in age-related maculopathy. *Ophthalmic Genet.* 2002;23:209-223.

30. Allikmets R. Further evidence for an association of ABCR alleles with age-related macular degeneration: the International ABCR Screening Consortium. *Am J Hum Genet.* 2000;67:487-491.

31. Stone EM, Braun TA, Russell SR, et al. Missense variations in the fibulin 5 gene and age-related macular degeneration. *N Engl J Med.* 2004;351:346-353.

32. Klein RJ, Zeiss C, Chew EY, et al. Complement factor H polymorphism in age-related macular degeneration. *Science.* 2005;308:385-389.

33. Haines JL, Hauser MA, Schmidt S, et al. Complement factor H variant increases the risk of age-related macular degeneration. *Science.* 2005;308:419-421.

34. Hageman GS, Anderson DH, Johnson LV, et al. A common haplotype in the complement regulatory gene factor H (HF1/CFH) predisposes individuals to age-related macular degeneration. *Proc Natl Acad Sci U S A.* 2005;102:7227-7232.

35. Edwards AO, Ritter R III, Abel KJ, Manning A, Panhuysen C, Farrer LA. Complement factor H polymorphism and age-related macular degeneration. *Science.* 2005;308:421-424.

36. Rivera A, Fisher SA, Fritsche LG, et al. Hypothetical LOC387715 is a second major susceptibility gene for age-related macular degeneration, contributing independently of complement factor H to disease risk. *Hum Mol Genet.* 2005;14:3227-3236.

37. Klein R, Myers CE, Meuer SM, et al. Risk alleles in CFH and ARMS2 and the long-term natural history of age-related macular degeneration: the Beaver Dam Eye Study. *JAMA Ophthalmol.* 2013;131:383-392.

38. Fritsche LG, Chen W, Schu M, et al. Seven new loci associated with age-related macular degeneration. *Nat Genet.* 2013;45:433-439, 439e1-2.

39. Chen W, Stambolian D, Edwards AO, et al. Genetic variants near TIMP3 and high-density lipoprotein-associated loci influence susceptibility to age-related macular degeneration. *Proc Natl Acad Sci U S A.* 2010;107:7401-7406.

40. Hageman GS, Hancox LS, Taiber AJ, et al. Extended haplotypes in the complement factor H (CFH) and CFH-related (CFHR) family of genes protect against age-related macular degeneration: characterization, ethnic distribution and evolutionary implications. *Ann Med.* 2006;38:592-604.

41. Heinen S, Hartmann A, Lauer N, et al. Factor H-related protein 1 (CFHR-1) inhibits complement C5 convertase activity and terminal complex formation. *Blood.* 2009;114:2439-2447.

42. Gold B, Merriam JE, Zernant J, et al. Variation in factor B (BF) and complement component 2 (C2) genes is associated with age-related macular degeneration. *Nat Genet.* 2006;38:458-462.

43. Jakobsdottir J, Conley YP, Weeks DE, Ferrell RE, Gorin MB. C2 and CFB genes in age-related maculopathy and joint action with CFH and LOC387715 genes. *PLoS One.* 2008;3:e2199.

44. Lee KY, Vithana EN, Mathur R, et al. Association analysis of CFH, C2, BF, and HTRA1 gene polymorphisms in Chinese patients with polypoidal choroidal vasculopathy. *Invest Ophthalmol Vis Sci.* 2008;49:2613-2619.

45. Despriet DD, van Duijn CM, Oostra BA, et al. Complement component C3 and risk of age-related macular degeneration. *Ophthalmology.* 2009;116:474-480.e2.

46. Spencer KL, Olson LM, Anderson BM, et al. C3 R102G polymorphism increases risk of age-related macular degeneration. *Hum Mol Genet.* 2008;17:1821-1824.

47. Seddon JM, Yu Y, Miller EC, et al. Rare variants in CFI, C3 and C9 are associated with high risk of advanced age-related macular degeneration. *Nat Genet.* 2013;45:1366-1370.

48. van de Ven JP, Nilsson SC, Tan PL, et al. A functional variant in the CFI gene confers a high risk of age-related macular degeneration. *Nat Genet.* 2013;45:813-817.

49. Zhang H, Morrison MA, Dewan A, et al. The NEI/NCBI dbGAP database: genotypes and haplotypes that may specifically predispose to risk of neovascular age-related macular degeneration. *BMC Med Genet.* 2008;9:51.

50. Conley YP, Jakobsdottir J, Mah T, et al. CFH, ELOVL4, PLEKHA1 and LOC387715 genes and susceptibility to age-related maculopathy: AREDS and CHS cohorts and meta-analyses. *Hum Mol Genet.* 2006;15:3206-3218.

51. Allikmets R, Dean M, Hageman GS, et al. The SERPING1 gene and age-related macular degeneration. *Lancet.* 2009;374:875-876.

52. Yang X, Hu J, Zhang J, Guan H. Polymorphisms in CFH, HTRA1 and CX3CR1 confer risk to exudative age-related macular degeneration in Han Chinese. *Br J Ophthalmol.* 2010;94:1211-1214.

53. Chen J, Connor KM, Smith LE. Overstaying their welcome: defective CX3CR1 microglia eyed in macular degeneration. *J Clin Invest.* 2007;117:2758-2762.

54. Chan CC, Tuo J, Bojanowski CM, Csaky KG, Green WR. Detection of CX3CR1 single nucleotide polymorphism and expression on archived eyes with age-related macular degeneration. *Histol Histopathol.* 2005;20:857-863.

55. Cho Y, Wang JJ, Chew EY, et al. Toll-like receptor polymorphisms and age-related macular degeneration: replication in three case-control samples. *Invest Ophthalmol Vis Sci.* 2009;50:5614-5618.

56. Edwards AO, Chen D, Fridley BL, et al. Toll-like receptor polymorphisms and age-related macular degeneration. *Invest Ophthalmol Vis Sci.* 2008;49:1652-1659.

57. Zareparsi S, Buraczynska M, Branham KE, et al. Toll-like receptor 4 variant D299G is associated with susceptibility to age-related macular degeneration. *Hum Mol Genet.* 2005;14:1449-1455.

58. Kanda A, Chen W, Othman M, et al. A variant of mitochondrial protein LOC387715/ARMS2,not HTRA1, is strongly associated with age-related macular degeneration. *Proc Natl Acad Sci U S A.* 2007;104(41):16227-16232.

59. Fuse N, Miyazawa A, Mengkegale M, et al. Polymorphisms in Complement Factor H and Hemicentin-1 genes in a Japanese population with dry-type age-related macular degeneration. *Am J Ophthalmol.* 2006;142:1074-1076.

60. Hayward C, Shu X, Cideciyan AV, et al. Mutation in a short-chain collagen gene, CTRP5, results in extracellular deposit formation in late-onset retinal degeneration: a genetic model for age-related macular degeneration. *Hum Mol Genet.* 2003;12:2657-2667.

61. Schultz DW, Klein ML, Humpert AJ, et al. Analysis of the ARMD1 locus: evidence that a mutation in HEMICENTIN-1 is associated with age-related macular degeneration in a large family. *Hum Mol Genet.* 2003;12:3315-3323.

62. Schultz DW, Weleber RG, Lawrence G, et al. HEMICENTIN-1 (FIBULIN-6) and the 1q31 AMD locus in the context of complex disease: review and perspective. *Ophthalmic Genet.* 2005;26:101-105.

63. Seitsonen S, Lemmela S, Holopainen J, et al. Analysis of variants in the complement factor H, the elongation of very long chain fatty acids-like 4 and the hemicentin 1 genes of age-related macular degeneration in the Finnish population. *Mol Vis.* 2006;12:796-801.

64. Thompson CL, Klein BE, Klein R, et al. Complement factor H and hemicentin-1 in age-related macular degeneration and renal phenotypes. *Hum Mol Genet.* 2007;16:2135-2148.

65. Miller JW. Age-related macular degeneration revisited—piecing the puzzle: the LXIX Edward Jackson memorial lecture. *Am J Ophthalmol.* 2013;155:1-35.e13.

66. van Driel MA, Maugeri A, Klevering BJ, Hoyng CB, Cremers FP. ABCR unites what ophthalmologists divide(s). *Ophthalmic Genet.* 1998;19(3):117-122.

67. Baum L, Chan WM, Li WY, Lam DS, Wang P, Pang CP. ABCA4 sequence variants in Chinese patients with age-related macular degeneration or Stargardt's disease. *Ophthalmologica.* 2003;(217):111-114.

68. Gibson J, Cree A, Collins A, Lotery A, Ennis S. Determination of a gene and environment risk model for age-related macular degeneration. *Br J Ophthalmol.* 2010;94:1382-1387.

69. Hagstrom SA, Ying GS, Pauer GJT, et al. Pharmacogenetics for genes associated with age-related macular degeneration in the Comparison of AMD Treatments Trials (CATT). *Ophthalmology.* 2013;120(3):593-599.

70. Seddon JM, Reynolds R, Yu Y, Daly MJ, Rosner B. Risk models for progression to advanced age-related macular degeneration using demographic, environmental, genetic, and ocular factors. *Ophthalmology.* 2011;118:2203-2211.

71. Chakravarthy U, Augood C, Bentham GC, et al. Cigarette smoking and age-related macular degeneration in the EUREYE Study. *Ophthalmology.* 2007;114:1157-1163.

72. Tomany SC, Wang JJ, Van Leeuwen R, et al. Risk factors for incident age-related macular degeneration: pooled findings from 3 continents. *Ophthalmology.* 2004;111:1280-1287.

73. Schmidt S, Hauser MA, Scott WK, et al. Cigarette smoking strongly modifies the association of LOC387715 and age-related macular degeneration. *Am J Hum Genet.* 2006;78:852-864.

74. Francis PJ, George S, Schultz DW, et al. The LOC387715 gene, smoking, body mass index, environmental associations with advanced age-related macular degeneration. *Hum Hered.* 2007;63:212-218.

75. Suner IJ, Espinosa-Heidmann DG, Marin-Castano ME, Hernandez EP, Pereira-Simon S, Cousins SW. Nicotine increases size and severity of experimental choroidal neovascularization. *Invest Ophthalmol Vis Sci.* 2004;45:311-317.

76. Alcazar O, Hawkridge AM, Collier TS, et al. Proteomics characterization of cell membrane blebs in human retinal pigment epithelium cells. *Mol Cell Proteomics.* 2009;8:2201-2211.

77. Age-Related Eye Disease Study Research Group. A randomized, placebo-controlled, clinical trial of high-dose supplementation with vitamins C and E, beta carotene, and zinc for age-related macular degeneration and vision loss: AREDS report no. 8. *Arch Ophthalmol.* 2001;119(10):1417-1436.

78. Seddon JM, Ajani UA, Sperduto RD, et al. Dietary carotenoids, vitamins A, C, and E, and advanced age-related macular degeneration. Eye Disease Case-Control Study Group. *JAMA.* 1994;272:1413-1420.

79. SanGiovanni JP, Chew EY, Agrón E, et al. The relationship of dietary omega-3 long-chain polyunsaturated fatty acid intake with incident age-related macular degeneration: AREDS report no. 23. *Arch Ophthalmol.* 2008;126:1274-1279.

80. Age-Related Eye Disease Study 2 Research Group. Lutein + zeaxanthin and omega-3 fatty acids for age-related macular degeneration: the Age-Related Eye Disease Study 2 (AREDS2) randomized clinical trial. *JAMA.* 2013;309:2005-2015.

81. Seddon JM, Reynolds R, Shah HR, Rosner B. Smoking, dietary betaine, methionine, and vitamin D in monozygotic twins with discordant macular degeneration: epigenetic implications. *Ophthalmology.* 2011;118:1386-1394.

82. Millen AE, Voland R, Sondel SA, et al. Vitamin D status and early age-related macular degeneration in postmenopausal women. *Arch Ophthalmol.* 2011;129:481-489.

83. Seddon JM, George S, Rosner B. Cigarette smoking, fish consumption, omega-3 fatty acid intake, and associations with age-related macular degeneration: the US Twin Study of Age-Related Macular Degeneration. *Arch Ophthalmol.* 2006;124:995-1001.

84. Delcourt C, Carriere I, Cristol JP, Lacroux A, Gerber M. Dietary fat and the risk of age-related maculopathy: the POLANUT study. *Eur J Clin Nutr.* 2007;61:1341–1344.

85. Cho E, Hung S, Willett WC, et al. Prospective study of dietary fat and the risk of age-related macular degeneration. *Am J Clin Nutr.* 2001;73:209-218.

86. Seddon JM, Rosner B, Sperduto RD, et al. Dietary fat and risk for advanced age-related macular degeneration. *Arch Ophthalmol.* 2001;119:1191-1199.

87. Seddon JM, Cote J, Rosner B. Progression of age-related macular degeneration: association with dietary fat, transunsaturated fat, nuts, and fish intake. *Arch Ophthalmol.* 2003;121:1728-1737.

88. Guymer RH, Chong EW. Modifiable risk factors for age-related macular degeneration. *Med J Aust.* 2006;184:455-458.

89. Robman L, Vu H, Hodge A, et al. Dietary lutein, zeaxanthin, and fats and the progression of age-related macular degeneration. *Can J Ophthalmol.* 2007;42:720-726.

90. Chong EW, Robman LD, Simpson JA, et al. Fat consumption and its association with age-related macular degeneration. *Arch Ophthalmol.* 2009;127:674-680.

91. Parekh N, Voland RP, Moeller SM, et al. Association between dietary fat intake and age-related macular degeneration in the Carotenoids in Age-Related Eye Disease Study (CAREDS): an ancillary study of the Women's Health Initiative. *Arch Ophthalmol.* 2009;127:1483-1493.

92. Dasari B, Prasanthi JR, Marwarha G, Singh BB, Ghribi O. Cholesterol-enriched diet causes age-related macular degeneration-like pathology in rabbit retina. *BMC Ophthalmol.* 2011;11:22.

93. Reynolds R, Rosner B, Seddon JM. Dietary omega-3 fatty acids, other fat intake, genetic susceptibility, and progression to incident geographic atrophy. *Ophthalmology.* 2013;120:1020-1080.

94. Seddon JM, Cote J, Davis N, Rosner B. Progression of age-related macular degeneration: association with body mass index, waist circumference, and waist-hip ratio. *Arch Ophthalmol.* 2003;121:785-792.

95. Comaschi M, Coscelli C, Cucinotta D, et al. Cardiovascular risk factors and metabolic control in type 2 diabetic subjects attending outpatient clinics in Italy: the SFIDA (survey of risk factors in Italian diabetic subjects by AMD) study. *Nutr Metab Cardiovasc Dis.* 2005;15:204-211.

96. Seddon JM, George S, Rosner B, Klein ML. CFH gene variant, Y402H, and smoking, body mass index, environmental associations with advanced age-related macular degeneration. *Hum Hered.* 2006;61:157-165.

97. Seddon JM, Reynolds R, Rosner B. Associations of smoking, body mass index, dietary lutein, and the LIPC gene variant rs10468017 with advanced age-related macular degeneration. *Mol Vis.* 2010;16:2412-2424.

98. Momeni-Moghaddam H, Kundart J, Ehsani M, Abdeh-Kykha A. Body mass index and binocular vision skills. *Saudi J Ophthalmol.* 2012;26:331-334.

99. Ulas F, Balbaba M, Ozmen S, Celebi S, Dogan U. Association of dehydroepiandrosterone sulfate, serum lipids, C-reactive protein and body mass index with age-related macular degeneration. *Int Ophthalmol.* 2013;33:485-491.

100. Snow KK, Seddon JM. Do age-related macular degeneration and cardiovascular disease share common antecedents? *Ophthalmic Epidemiol.* 1999;6:125-143.

101. Sui GY, Liu GC, Liu GY, et al. Is sunlight exposure a risk factor for age-related macular degeneration? A systematic review and meta-analysis. *Br J Ophthalmol.* 2013;97:389-394.

102. Smith W, Assink J, Klein R, et al. Risk factors for age-related macular degeneration: pooled findings from three continents. *Ophthalmology.* 2001;108:697-704.

103. Chakravarthy U, Wong TY, Fletcher A, et al. Clinical risk factors for age-related macular degeneration: a systematic review and meta-analysis. *BMC Ophthalmol.* 2010;10:31.

104. Cugati S, Mitchell P, Rochtchina E, Tan AG, Smith W, Wang JJ. Cataract surgery and the 10-year incidence of age-related maculopathy: the Blue Mountains Eye Study. *Ophthalmology.* 2006;113:2020-2025.

105. Sandberg MA, Tolentino MJ, Miller S, Berson EL, Gaudio AR. Hyperopia and neovascularization in age-related macular degeneration. *Ophthalmology.* 1993;100:1009-1013.

106. Chew EY, Sperduto RD, Milton RC, et al. Risk of advanced age-related macular degeneration after cataract surgery in the Age-Related Eye Disease Study: AREDS report 25. *Ophthalmology.* 2009;116:297-303.

2

PATHOLOGY OF AGE-RELATED MACULAR DEGENERATION

Nora M.V. Laver, MD

This chapter discusses the normal function of and interactions among the photoreceptors, the retinal pigment epithelium (RPE), Bruch's membrane, and the choriocapillaris. It also discusses the normal age-related changes found in these structures and compares the pathological changes that undermine the normal function, leading to AMD.[1]

NORMAL HISTOPATHOLOGY FEATURES

Photoreceptors

The photoreceptors convert light into signals that stimulate neuronal impulse transmission to the cerebral cortex, which are ultimately interpreted as vision. The rods are narrower than the cones and are much more sensitive to light, whereas the cones are less sensitive but respond to a narrower range of wavelengths (hence they sense color). In the macular region, the fovea is dominated by cones, whereas the surrounding paramacular region is rod dominated (Figure 2-1).

The photoreceptor inner segments are rich in mitochondria, which are needed to provide energy. The outer segments contain closely packed discs containing opsins, molecules that absorb photons, combined with a pigment molecule called retinal; these compounds are called *rhodopsin* in rods and *photopsins* in cones. The key initial step in the visual cycle happens when a photon of light hits the photoreceptor outer segment, causing conversion of 11-*cis*-retinal to its isomer all-*trans*-retinal, leading to a signal cascade and hyperpolarization of the photoreceptor cell. All-*trans*-retinal is then reduced and travels to the RPE, where it is converted back to 11-*cis*-retinal and transferred back to the photoreceptor outer segment, so the visual cycle may repeat itself.[1]

Retinal Pigment Epithelium

The RPE is a single layer of hexagonal cells that are packed with melanin pigment. It is firmly attached to its basement membrane, and each cell contains an oval

Duker JS, Witkin AJ, eds.
Age-Related Macular Degeneration:
Current Management (pp. 15-29)
© 2015 Taylor & Francis Group

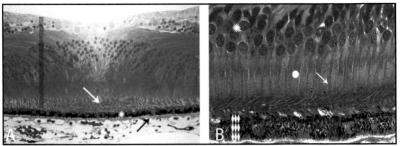

Figure 2-1. (A) Toloudine blue staining of human macula and fovea (dashed lines) with cones (white arrow), RPE (white asterisk), and Bruch's membrane (black arrow) (original magnification ×20). (B) Richardson's mixture stain showing parafoveal cones (white circle=photoreceptor outer segment; white asterisk=photoreceptor nuclei), fewer rods (white arrow), and RPE (white diamonds) (original magnification ×63). (Reprinted with permission from Milam AH, John SK. Human Retina Teaching Set. Philadelphia, PA: Scheie Eye Institute, University of Pennsylvania. http://www.uphs.upenn.edu/ophthalmology/education/teachingset.htm.)

nucleus with an anterior portion extending in a series of finger-like processes that interdigitate with the photoreceptor outer segments. The RPE cells have numerous infoldings of the cell membrane along the basal border of the cells and are separated from the underlying basement membrane by a small space (Figure 2-2). The cells contain numerous melanosomes, melanin granules, golgi complexes, lysosomes, rough and smooth endoplasmic reticulum, and mitochondria.

The RPE provides nutrients, such as glucose and omega-3 fatty acids, to the photoreceptor outer segments, and it transports water, ions, and metabolic end products from the subretinal space to the choroid. RPE melanosomes absorb excess incoming light to prevent retinal light damage. It is involved in the phagocytosis of shed outer segments of the photoreceptors, in addition to playing a key role in forming the outer blood-retinal barrier. The RPE produces and secretes numerous growth factors, including vascular endothelial growth factor (VEGF) and pigment epithelium-derived factor.[2,3]

Bruch's Membrane

Bruch's membrane is a stratified extracellular matrix complex, 1 to 4 μm thick, located between the RPE and the choriocapillaris. In healthy individuals, it has a pentalaminar structure under transmission electron microscopy (EM). It is composed of the following (see Figure 2-2):

1. The basement membrane of the RPE (0.14 to 0.15 μm thick)
2. An inner collagenous layer (1.4 μm in diameter)
3. A middle elastic layer
4. An outer collagenous layer (0.7 μm thick)
5. The basement membrane of the endothelium of the choriocapillaris[4]

The inner and outer collagenous zones show interlacing patterns and communicate with each other through the middle elastic layer. The elastic layer of Bruch's membrane is 3 to 6 times thinner and 2 to 5 times more porous in the macular region than it is in the peripheral regions in all ages.[5]

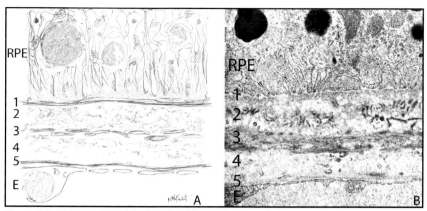

Figure 2-2. (A) Illustration of the RPE, Bruch's membrane, and choriocapillaris complex, similar to the electron microscopy features in shown in Figure 2-2B. (Drawing by Nada Farhat, MD, MPH.) (B) Electron microscopy of pentalaminar Bruch's membrane composed of (1) the basement membrane of the RPE, (2) inner collagenous layer, (3) middle elastic layer, (4) outer collagenous layer, and (5) the basement membrane of the endothelium of the choriocapillaris (original magnification ×6000). Abbreviations: E, endothelium of the choriocapillaris; RPE, retinal pigment epithelium.

The main components of Bruch's membrane are collagens type I, III, IV, V, and VI[6]; fibronectin; laminin; heparin sulphate proteoglycans; and chondroitin/dermatan sulphate.[7-9] Bruch's membrane functions as a physical and biochemical barrier in normal physiological states. Bruch's membrane most likely provides a scaffold for RPE adhesion, regulates the diffusion of molecules between the choroid and retina, and serves as a physical barrier to cell movement, restricting the passage of cells between the choroid and retina.[4]

Choriocapillaris

The choriocapillaris is arranged in a single layer and localized in the anterior portion of the choroid, closest to the RPE and the retina (see Figure 2-2). Feeding arterioles and draining venules enter the capillary bed at right angles from below. The choriocapillaris is composed of fenestrated endothelial cells enveloped by a basement membrane, presenting a single-layer cell membrane that interfaces with Bruch's membrane. Red blood cells are present in the lumens of the choroidal capillaries, and melanocytic cells are observed in the stroma. Normal choroidal capillaries are known to extend cellular processes through their basal lamina, and these processes are thought to anchor and stabilize the choriocapillaris. The vascular cells are reported to express VEGF receptor 1 and 2 and intracellular adhesion molecule 1 (ICAM-1), which are needed for firm adhesion of activated neutrophils.[10]

AGING HISTOPATHOLOGICAL CHANGES

The macula is one of the most metabolically active parts of the body. This, along with continuous light exposure and the presence of photoactivated molecules, leads to creation of an enormous amount of potentially damaging reactive oxygen species. Oxidative damage is minimized by a variety of free radical–absorbing pigments and compounds

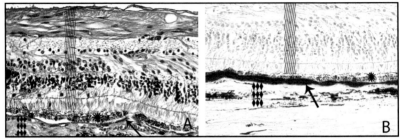

Figure 2-3. (A) Hematoxylin-eosin staining of thickened and fragmented Bruch's membrane due to aging (back arrow), RPE (black asterisk), choriocapillaris (black diamonds), and retina (black dashed lines) in a 92-year-old man (original magnification ×4). (B) Azarine red calcium staining of Bruch's membrane (black arrow), RPE (black asterisk), choriocapillaris (black diamonds), and retina (black dashed lines) in normal aging (original magnification ×4).

and molecular repair systems; however, over time, oxidative damage occurs to a variety of structures of the macula, ultimately leading to many of the age-related changes described here.[11]

Localized and diffuse thickening of the inner aspect of Bruch's membrane is one of the key changes that occurs with aging. This thickening is mainly composed of widely spaced collagen and abnormal basement membrane deposits, referred to as basal laminar deposits, or BLamD,[12] and granular material containing coated and noncoated vesicles and phospholipids, referred to as basal linear deposits, or BLinD. In addition, enhanced sudanophilia due to lipid deposits decreases in hydraulic conductivity, and fragmentation and calcification of Bruch's membrane are also found with aging (Figure 2-3). The density and diameters of the choriocapillaris vessels also decrease with age (Figure 2-4).[11]

Decreased Macular Elastic Layer Integrity

Pathological features occurring in AMD include changes in the structural integrity of Bruch's elastic middle layer around the macula.[4] The integrity of the macular elastic layer is significantly lower in individuals with early-stage AMD. In late-stage AMD, including those with active choroidal neovascularization (CNV) and disciform scars (discussed later in the chapter), thickness and integrity of the elastic layer are both significantly lower. The less porous macular elastic layer might lead to less substrate for RPE cell adhesion and less propensity for pigment epithelial cell detachments and dysfunction of macular RPE cells. Inflammatory and immune-mediated processes, particularly complement activation (see Chapter 1), are prominent at the macular RPE/Bruch's membrane interphase region. Consequently, disruption, degradation, and/or remodeling of Bruch's membrane–associated elastin and collagen may occur (Figure 2-5).[4]

Basal Laminar Deposits and Basal Linear Deposits

BLamD are found between the RPE cytoplasmic membrane and the basal lamina of the RPE. They are found in histologic examinations and are almost invisible clinically.[12-14] BLamD consist of basement membrane material and long-spaced collagen (Figure 2-6). Two types of BLamD have been described: early and late. BLamD thickness correlates well with the degree of RPE degeneration, photoreceptor fallout, and vision loss. A late, amorphous form of BLamD is associated with more severe RPE degeneration.

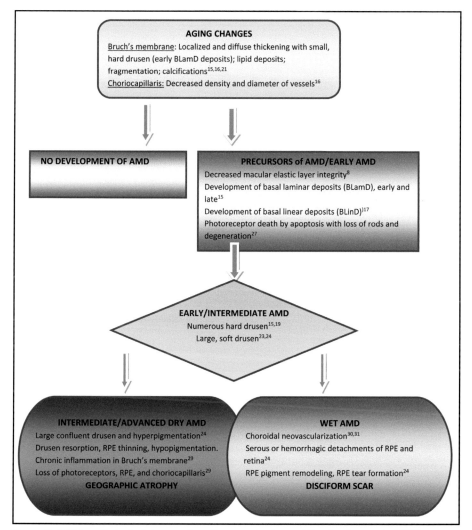

Figure 2-4. Histopathological changes found in normal aging and the development of AMD.

BLinD consist of vesicular material and are localized between the basal lamina of the RPE and the inner collagenous layer of Bruch's membrane.[14] BLinD are composed of membranous bodies released from the basal plasma membrane of the RPE that are unable to enter the inner collagenous layer, which is the layer that imparts the major resistance to fluid movement. These deposits are periodic acid-Schiff stain positive and have high lipid content.

A threshold of early AMD is the presence of both BLinD and continuous early BLamD (see Figure 2-6).[14] The accumulation of late BLamD correlates with increasing BLamD thickness, advancing RPE degeneration, poorer vision, increasing age, and clinically evident pigment changes. When produced, BLamD is resilient, persisting even in areas of geographic atrophy and disciform scars. BLamD and membranous debris may be the

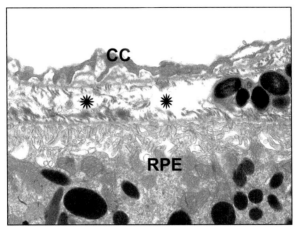

Figure 2-5. Electron microscopy of RPE/Bruch's membrane interphase shows disruption and degradation of Bruch's membrane–associated elastin and collagen (black asterisks) (original magnification ×6000). Abbreviation: CC, choriocapillaris. (Reprinted with permission from Gendron RL, Laver NV, Good WV, et al. Loss of tubedown expression as a contributing factor in the development of age-related retinopathy. *Inv Ophthalmol Vis Sci.* 2010;51[10]:5267-5277.)

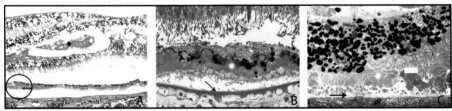

Figure 2-6. (A) Hematoxylin-eosin staining of basal laminar deposits (white arrow in circle) and basal linear deposits (black arrow in circle) in the retina of a 76-year-old man with AMD and cystoid macular edema (black asterisk) (original magnification ×10). (B) Toloudine blue staining of BLamD (white asterisk) between the RPE and Bruch's membrane (black arrow) in a patient with advanced AMD (original magnification ×100). (Reprinted with permission from Hagerman G. Age-related macular degeneration [AMD]. In: Kolb H, Nelson R, Fernandez E, Jones B, eds. *Webvision: The Organization of the Retina and Visual System.* Salt Lake City, UT: University of Utah Health Sciences Center. http://webvision.med.utah.edu.) (C) Electron microscopy of BLamD (white asterisk) accumulated between the basal surface of the RPE (white rectangle) and its basal lamina (black arrow) (original magnification ×1500). (Reprinted with permission from Hagerman G. Age-related macular degeneration [AMD]. In: Kolb H, Nelson R, Fernandez E, Jones B, eds. *Webvision: The Organization of the Retina and Visual System.* Salt Lake City, UT: University of Utah Health Sciences Center. http://webvision.med.utah.edu.)

products of cell survival strategies of RPE under stress. Early BLamD can be thought of as an excess basement membrane secreted by the RPE, a strategy used by cells attempting to recover from injury, allowing them to remain attached to a tissue's scaffolding. As BLamD thickens, the deposits separate the basal RPE surface from its original basement membrane and choroidal blood supply, thus decreasing the permeability of Bruch's membrane.[14,15] The production of late BLamD signals a critical RPE damage point at which the secreted basement membrane material becomes more condensed and the RPE cells become hyperpigmented, enlarged, lose their microvilli, and round off and are thus no longer able to support the photoreceptors. They eventually lose their anchoring to both the basement membrane and to adjacent cells and are shed into the subretinal space.[1,14,15]

Epidemiological data show that eyes with a large amount of membranous debris in the form of large drusen are at the highest risk of developing advanced AMD over a 5- to 10-year period.[16] Eyes with pigment changes alone are at a lower risk of developing advanced AMD over the same period of time, suggesting an alternate slower disease course.

DRUSEN

Drusen represent the first clinically visible changes in the ocular fundus (see Figure 2-4), but they are not uniquely associated with AMD. Drusen appear as yellowish-white dots in the macula, the paramacular area, and the retinal periphery. AMD is associated with 2 types of drusen, which have different clinical appearances and different prognoses.[17]

Hard Drusen

Hard drusen appear as small yellow nodules with discreet margins (Figure 2-7). They consist of hyaline material, similar to hyalinized Bruch's membrane, and have an amorphous appearance on electron microscopy. They may be present at any age. Numerous hard drusen are an independent risk factor for vision loss in AMD.[12,16]

Hard drusen have been identified in the macula in 83% of postmortem eyes.[13,18] Drusen develop by entrapment of unwanted basal cytoplasm through the basement membrane of the RPE by a process similar to apoptosis—a process of evagination and pinching off of cytoplasm from the base of the RPE. These entrapment sites are found at all ages, indicating a normal aging phenomenon.[18]

In eyes with many small, hard drusen, Bruch's membrane is thicker, appearing as a row of microdrusen or rounded elevations 2 μm in diameter and composed of dense amorphous material. All drusen types may disappear in time, but these areas of drusen may be replaced by more severe manifestations of AMD.

Soft Drusen

Soft drusen are larger (>63 μm) granular amorphous vesicular structures with indistinct edges (Figure 2-8). Several types of soft drusen have been observed and include localized detachment of BLamD, with or without BLinD. Soft drusen tend to become confluent, which is an independent risk factor for AMD.[17] Multiple and confluent soft drusen can create large RPE detachments and often lead to CNV formation.

Longitudinal clinical studies of at least 5 years' duration suggest that advanced AMD rarely develops in eyes with small, hard drusen only, regardless of the total area involved.[19] Drusen characteristics that correlate with progression to exudative maculopathy include 5 or more drusen, drusen >63 μm in size, and a confluence of drusen (see Chapter 3).[20]

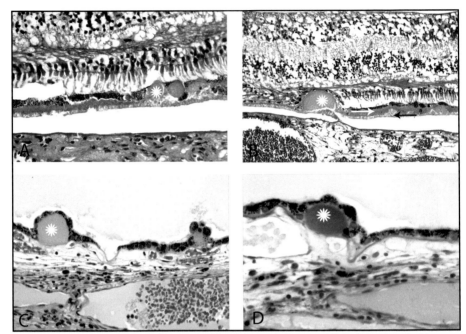

Figure 2-7. (A) Periodic acid-Schiff staining of hard drusen (white asterisk) in the retina of a 76-year-old man with AMD (original magnification ×20). (B) Periodic acid-Schiff staining of hard drusen (white asterisk) seen in association with BLamD (white arrow) and BLinD (black arrow) deposits in Bruch's membrane in the retina of a 76-year-old man with AMD (original magnification ×10). (C) Hematoxylin-eosin staining and (D) periodic acid-Schiff staining of hard drusen (white asterisks) in the retina of an 86-year-old woman with early AMD (original magnification ×20).

Drusen Composition

Histologically, drusen are composed of granular ground substance, degenerating lipid and protein particles, crystalline deposits of calcium and amino acids, residual bodies, and partially digested photoreceptor outer segment discs.

Components of the complement system, including C3 complement fragments, C5, and the membrane-attack complex (C5b-9), have been shown to be present in drusen.[2,21] Dysregulation of complement leads to overactive complement activity that can cause immune-mediated damage. A polymorphism in complement factor H, a key regulator of complement activation, has been identified as a major risk factor for the development of AMD (see Chapter 1).[22]

Drusen formation shares similarities with amyloid diseases, such as Alzheimer's disease and Parkinson's disease. Although amyloid proteins, such as the Aβ peptide, transthyretin, immunoglobulin light chains, and amyloid A, are found in drusen and sub-RPE deposits, nonfibrillar oligomers, rather than amyloid fibrils, appear to be the primary toxic agents present centrally within drusen and in close proximity to the inner collagenous layer of Bruch's membrane.[23] Antigen-presenting dendritic cells are present in and around drusen and may facilitate the clearance of amyloid oligomers.

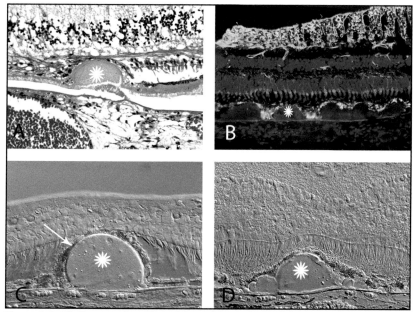

Figure 2-8. (A) Hematoxylin-eosin staining of large drusen (white asterisk) in the retina of a 76-year-old man with AMD (original magnification ×40). (B) Confluent drusen near the optic nerve head (white asterisk). Astrocytes are seen (green) that are positive for glial fibrillary acidic protein in the nerve fiber layer. The cones (red; mAb 7G6) are decreased in number, and their outer segments are shortened over drusen. Cell nuclei are stained blue (4',6-diamidino-2-phenylindole). The RPE shows areas of thinning and depigmentation (original magnification ×20). (Reprinted with permission from Milam AH, John SK. Human Retina Teaching Set. Philadelphia, PA: Scheie Eye Institute, University of Pennsylvania.   http://www.uphs.upenn.edu/ophthalmology/education/teachingset.htm.) (C) Electron microscopy with Nomarski optics shows giant drusen (white asterisk) with cell nuclei stained lavender (original magnification ×63). The RPE overlying the giant drusen is thinned and shows depigmentation (white arrow). (Reprinted with permission from Milam AH, John SK. Human Retina Teaching Set. Philadelphia, PA: Scheie Eye Institute, University of Pennsylvania. http://www.uphs.upenn.edu/ophthalmology/education/teachingset.htm.) (D) Electron microscopy with Nomarski optics shows confluent drusen (white asterisk) with RPE thinning and depigmentation (original magnification ×40). (Reprinted with permission from Milam AH, John SK. Human Retina Teaching Set. Philadelphia, PA: Scheie Eye Institute, University of Pennsylvania. http://www.uphs.upenn.edu/ophthalmology/education/teachingset.htm.)

RETINAL PIGMENT EPITHELIUM CHANGES LEADING TO ATROPHY

It has been suggested that photoreceptor death by apoptosis starts early in AMD.[24] In non-neovascular (dry) AMD, typical findings are pigment disruption and drusen. Large, confluent drusen formation and hyperpigmentation due to RPE dysfunction (see Figure 2-4) are the initial insults leading to resorption of these drusen and loss of RPE with hypopigmentation (see Figure 2-8). Incipient atrophy is a stage that immediately precedes geographic atrophy. Areas of RPE thinning or depigmentation can be recognized (Figure 2-9). The retina appears pinker and drusen appear whiter and harder before fading. Multinucleated giant cells and mononuclear inflammatory cells are observed

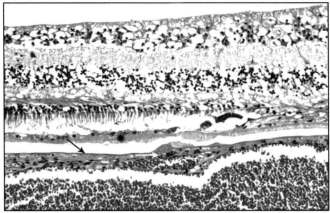

Figure 2-9. Hematoxylin-eosin staining of choroidal neovascularization (white arrow) in the sub-RPE space of a 76-year-old man with AMD. Basal laminar deposits (black asterisk) and Bruch's membrane (black arrow) are also shown (original magnification ×10).

lying on Bruch's membrane at the margin of areas of geographic atrophy and may play a role in clearing the debris from the necrotic cells at this site.[25,26]

In expanding areas of atrophy, the junctional zone lipofuscin content of the RPE is maximal, presumably due to both autophagy and outer-segment phagocytosis and engulfment of discarded RPE and their photoreceptor cells. The surviving photoreceptors are abnormal cones, with widened inner segments and absent outer segments, with no evidence of phagocytosis. The photoreceptors and RPE then disappear together. Within the area of atrophy, there is absence of photoreceptors, RPE, and choriocapillaris. The outer nuclear layer of the retina disappears, causing the outer plexiform layer to rest directly on Bruch's membrane. When there is loss of RPE and photoreceptors, the basal linear deposits disappear. Obliteration of the choriocapillaris is followed by erosion of the intercapillary pillars of Bruch's membrane and, in long-standing cases, the membrane becomes thinner.

CHOROIDAL NEOVASCULARIZATION TYPES 1, 2, AND 3

Neovascular (wet) AMD implies that fluid, exudates, and/or blood vessels are present in the extracellular space between the neural retina and the RPE, and/or between the RPE and Bruch's membrane. The neovascular tissue associated with exudative AMD is referred to as CNV (see Figure 2-4) because it typically originates from the choriocapillaris and extends through a dehiscence in Bruch's membrane into the subretinal or sub-RPE space (Figure 2-10).[20,27]

Ingrowth of new vessels from the choriocapillaris into the sub-RPE space, associated with damage to the outer retina, is called *neovascularization type 1* (Figure 2-11). When the growth is into the subretinal space, it is termed *neovascularization type 2*. Retinal angiomatous proliferation—a distinct form, termed *type 3 neovascularization*—may originate not only from the choroid but also from deep retinal capillaries.[28]

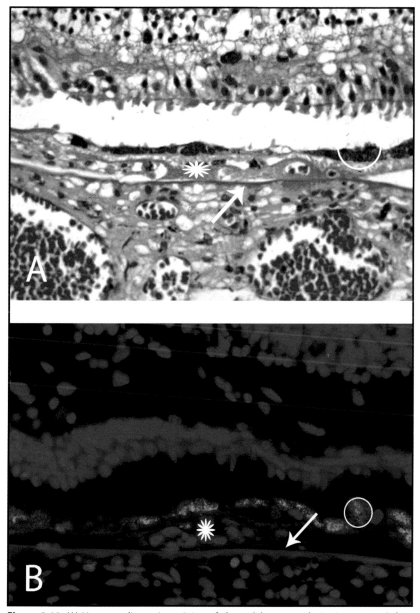

Figure 2-10. (A) Hematoxylin-eosin staining of choroidal neovascularization type 1 (white asterisk) in the macula of a 76-year-old man with AMD present between Bruch's membrane (white arrow) and the RPE (white circle) (original magnification ×20). (B) Choroidal neovascularization type 1 (white asterisk), RPE (white circle), and Bruch's membrane (white arrow). Cell nuclei are stained blue (4',6-diamidino-2-phenylindole), and RPE cells are stained orange (original magnification ×20). (Reprinted with permission from Milam AH, John SK. Human Retina Teaching Set. Philadelphia, PA: Scheie Eye Institute, University of Pennsylvania. http://www.uphs.upenn.edu/ophthalmology/education/teachingset.htm.)

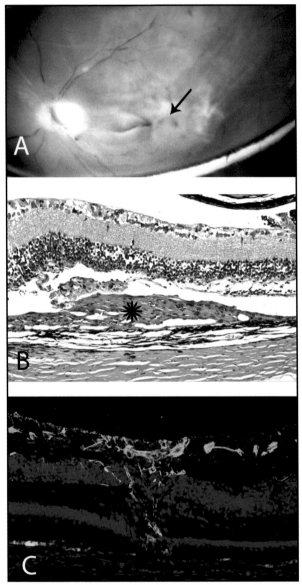

Figure 2-11. (A) Low-power view on gross examination of the mac-ula (black arrow) of a 76-year-old man with wet AMD (original mag-nification ×1). (B) Hematoxylin-eosin staining of disciform scar in the sub-RPE space (black asterisk) in a 90-year-old-woman with late AMD (original magnification ×10). (C) Area of geographic atrophy with reactive Müller cells seen in green (anti-glial fibrillary acidic protein), filling the area of lost photoreceptors. Cell nuclei are stained blue (4',6-diamidino-2-phenylindole), and RPE cells are stained orange (original magnification ×20). (Reprinted with permission from Milam AH, John SK. Human Retina Teaching Set. Philadelphia, PA: Scheie Eye Institute, University of Pennsylvania. http://www.uphs.upenn.edu/ophthalmology/education/teachingset.htm.)

In the early stages of AMD, the vessels are capillary like; over time they evolve into arteries and veins. CNV may lead to serous and/or hemorrhagic detachments of the RPE and retina, pigment modeling, exudation, and RPE tears.[29]

CNV is considered a wound-healing response to an RPE insult. An RPE protein (pigment epithelium-derived factor) has an inhibitory effect on ocular neovascularization. VEGF, a well-known angiogenic factor, may be produced by endothelial cells, pericytes, glial cells, Müller cells, ganglion cells, photoreceptors, and RPE. The growth of CNV is determined by the balance between antiangiogenic and angiogenic factors. The cause of increased VEGF in eyes with CNV is not clear, but it is typically overexpressed in tissues with hypoxia, high glucose and protein C activation, advanced glycation end products, reactive oxygen species, activated oncogenes, and various cytokines.

Histopathological studies of CNV from submacular surgery specimens have demonstrated the presence of VEGF. In CNV, both angiogenesis (growth of new vessels from preexisting vessels) and vasculogenesis (de novo growth of blood vessels) occur. Up to 20% of endothelial cells are bone marrow–derived progenitor cells, which join the activated resident endothelial cells to form the new vascular structures. Integrins and metalloproteinases are important for migration of endothelial cells and remodeling of extracellular matrix to allow CNV infiltration through Bruch's membrane.[29-31] Platelet-derived growth factor recruits pericytes to the new vessels to achieve vascular maturation. Insults to the structural integrity of the elastic layer of Bruch's membrane lead to invasion of CNV into the sub-RPE or subretinal spaces.

DEVELOPMENT OF DISCIFORM SCARRING

Left untreated, the natural history of neovascular AMD advances further to a cicatricial stage, called a disciform scar. Scars may be vascularized or nonvascularized (see Figure 2-11).[31] Scars are located between BLamD and the remainder of Bruch's membrane or in the sub-RPE space, with BLinD underlying the macula, accompanied by a central scotoma with central vision loss. Disciform scars are composed primarily of fibrous tissue, as compared with active CNV lesions, which have both fibrous and vascular components.

SUMMARY

The normal relationship within the photoreceptors, RPE, Bruch's membrane, and the choriocapillaris is lost in wet and dry AMD, resulting in death and dysfunction of all of the components. The various histopathological changes of AMD are a continuum from the development of basal deposits, RPE attenuation, depigmentation, hyperplasia, atrophy, soft drusen formation, development of choroidal neovascularization, and formation of a disciform scar.

ACKNOWLEDGMENT

Special thanks to Nada Farhat, MD, MPH for her contribution of the illustration of the RPE, Bruch's membrane, and choriocapillaris complex shown in Figure 2-1A.

REFERENCES

1. Palczewski K. Chemistry and biology of vision. *J Biol Chem.* 2012;287(3):1612-1619.
2. Adamis AP, Shima DT, Yeo KT, et al. Synthesis and secretion of vascular permeability factor/vascular endothelial growth factor by human retinal pigment epithelial cells. *Biochem Biophys Res Commun.* 1993;193(2):631-638.
3. Blaauwgeers HG, Holtkamp GM, Rutten H, et al. Polarized vascular endothelial growth factor secretion by human retinal pigment epithelium and localization of vascular endothelial growth factor receptors on the inner choriocapillaris: evidence for a trophic paracrine relation. *Am J Pathol.* 1999;155(2):421-428.
4. Bhutto I, Lutty G. Understanding age-related macular degeneration (AMD): relationships between the photoreceptor/retinal pigment epithelium/Bruch's membrane/choriocapillaris complex. *Mol Aspects Med.* 2012;33(4):295-317.
5. Chong NHV, Keonin J, Luthert PJ et al. Decreased thickness and integrity of the macular elastic layer of Bruch's membrane correspond to the distribution of lesions associated with age-related macular degeneration. *Am J Pathol.* 2005;166(1):214-251.
6. Chen L, Miyamura N, Ninomiya Y, Handa JT. Distribution of the collagen IV isoforms in human Bruch's membrane. *Br J Ophthalmol.* 2003;87(2):212-215.
7. Pauleikhoff D, Zuels S, Sheraidah GS, Marshall J, Wessing A, Bird AC. Correlation between biochemical composition and fluorescein binding of deposits in Bruch's membrane. *Ophthalmology.* 1992;99(10):1548-1553.
8. Aisenbrey S, Zhang M, Bacher D, Yee J, Brunken WJ, Hunter DD. Retinal pigment epithelial cells synthesize laminins, including laminin 5, and adhere to them through alpha3- and alpha6-containing integrins. *Invest Ophthalmol Vis Sci.* 2006;47(12):5537-5544.
9. Hewitt AT, Nakazawa K, Newsome DA. Analysis of newly synthesized Bruch's membrane proteoglycans. *Invest Ophthalmol Vis Sci.* 1989;30(3):478-486.
10. Hogan MJ. Ultrastructure of the choroid: its role in the pathogenesis of chorioretinal diseases. *Trans Pac Coast Otoophthalmol Soc Annu Meet.* 1961;42:61-87.
11. Jarrett SG1, Boulton ME. Consequences of oxidative stress in age-related macular degeneration. *Mol Aspects Med.* 2012;33(4):399-417.
12. Sarks S, Cherepanoff S, Killingsworth M, Sarks J. Relationship of basal laminar deposit and membranous debris to the clinical presentation of early age-related macular degeneration. *Inv Ophthalm Vis Sci.* 2007;48(3):968-977.
13. Green WR, Enger C. Age-related macular degeneration histopathologic studies; the 1992 Lorenz E. Zimmerman lecture. *Ophthalmology.* 1993;100:1519-1535.
14. Curcio C, Millican C. Basal linear deposit and large drusen are specific for early age-related maculopathy. *Arch Ophthalmol.* 1999;117:329-339.
15. Binder S, Falkner-Radler CI. Age-related macular degeneration I: types and future directions. In: Cavallotti CA, Cerulli L, eds. *Age-Related Changes of the Human Eye.* Totowa, NJ: Humana Press; 2008:239-256.
16. Bird AC, Bressler NM, Bressler SB, et al. An international classification and grading system for age-related maculopathy and age-related macular degeneration. The International ARM Epidemiological Study Group. *Surv Ophthalmol.* 1995;39(5):367-374.
17. Abdelsalam A, Zarbin MA. Review of drusen pathogenesis, natural history and laser photocoaguation-induced regression in age-related macular degeneration. *Surv Ophthalmol.* 1999;44(1):1-29.
18. Spraul CW, Grossniklaus HE. Characteristics of drusen and Bruch's membrane in postmortem eyes with age-related macular degeneration. *Arch Ophthalmol.* 1997;115(2):267-273.
19. Age-Related Eye Disease Study Research Group. A randomized, placebo-controlled, clinical trial of high-dose supplementation with vitamins C and E, beta carotene, and zinc for age-related macular degeneration and vision loss: AREDS report no. 8. *Arch Ophthalmol.* 2001;119:1417-1436.
20. van der Schaft TL, Mooy CM, de Bruijn WC, Oron FG, Mulder PG, de Jong PT. Histologic features of the early stages of age-related macular degeneration: a statistical analysis. *Ophthalmology.* 1992;99:278-286.

21. Jager RD, Mieler WF, Miller JW. Age-related macular degeneration. *N Engl J Med.* 2008;358(24):2606-2617.

22. Hageman GS, Anderson DH, Johnson LV, et al. A common haplotype in the complement regulatory gene factor H (HF1/CFH) predisposes individuals to age related macular degeneration. *Proc Natl Acad Sci U S A.* 2005;102(20):7227-7232.

23. Luibl V, Isas JM, Kayed R, Glabe CG, Langen R, Chen J. Drusen deposits associated with aging and age-related macular degeneration contain nonfibrillar amyloid oligomers. *J Clin Invest.* 2006;116(2):378-385.

24. Curcio CA, Medeiros NE, Millican CL. Photoreceptor loss in age-related macular degeneration. *Invest Ophthal Vis Sci.* 1996;37:1236-1249.

25. Ferris FL, Davis MD, Clemons TE, et al. A simplified severity scale for age-related macular degeneration: AREDS report no. 18. *Arch Ophthalmol.* 2005;123(11):1570-1574.

26. Green RW. Histopathology of age-related macular degeneration. *Mol Vis.* 1999;5:27.

27. Grossniklaus HE, Green WR. Choroidal neovascularization. *Am J Ophthalmol.* 2004;137(3):496-503.

28. Grossniklaus HE, Martinez JA, Brown VB, et al. Immunohistochemical and histochemical properties of surgically excised subretinal neovascular membranes in age-related macular degeneration. *Am J Ophthalmol.* 1992;114(4):464-472.

29. Espinosa-Heidmann DG, Caicedo A, Hernandez EP, Csaky KG, Cousins SW. Bone marrow-derived progenitor cells contribute to experimental choroidal neovascularization. *Invest Ophthalmol Vis Sci.* 2003;44(11):4914-4919.

30. Sengupta N, Caballero S, Mames RN, Timmers AM, Saban D, Grant MB. Preventing stem cell incorporation into choroidal neovascularization by targeting homing and attachment factors. *Invest Ophthalmol Vis Sci.* 2005;46(1):343-348.

31. Tomita M, Yamada H, Adachi Y, Cui Y, Yamada E, Higuchi A. Choroidal neovascularization is provided by bone marrow cells. *Stem Cells.* 2004;22(1):21-26.

3

CLINICAL DIAGNOSIS, CLASSIFICATION, AND PATIENT COUNSELING

Sana Nadeem, MBBS and Nadia K. Waheed, MD, MPH

Age-related macular degeneration (AMD) is routinely diagnosed based on the identification of characteristic clinical findings. Classification of AMD can be helpful to determine a risk stratification of each patient. AMD is routinely divided into 2 forms:

1. Non-neovascular (atrophic, dry)

2. Neovascular (exudative, wet)

Characteristics of dry AMD include the presence of drusen, retinal pigment epithelium (RPE) clumping, areas of RPE hypopigmentation, and, in the more advanced stage, geographic atrophy (GA) (Figures 3-1 and 3-2). Wet AMD is characterized by the presence of choroidal neovascularization (CNV) in the macula, which may lead to hemorrhage, fluid and/or exudate accumulation, and disciform scarring in the late stage. In patients with dry AMD, characteristics identified on examination can help predict the risk of progression of AMD. A higher risk of progression is associated with a larger number of drusen (>5); larger-sized drusen (>63 μm); soft, indistinct, and/or confluent drusen; pigment abnormalities; and/or the presence of advanced AMD (GA or CNV) in the fellow eye.[1-4]

This chapter will focus primarily on components of the clinical examination that aid in diagnosis and management of AMD, characterization of the different types of AMD, and some important aspects of patient counseling that retina physicians perform on a daily basis. Key risk factor assessments, such as family history, nutrition, cardiovascular risk factors, and smoking history, as well as genetic testing, were discussed in Chapter 1. Treatment paradigms for the management of wet AMD, an ever-expanding field, are also discussed later in this book.

SYMPTOMS OF AGE-RELATED MACULAR DEGENERATION

AMD is frequently asymptomatic in its early forms and is detected only on routine ocular fundus examination. Common presenting symptoms include blurred central

Duker JS, Witkin AJ, eds.
Age-Related Macular Degeneration:
Current Management (pp. 31-42)
© 2015 Taylor & Francis Group

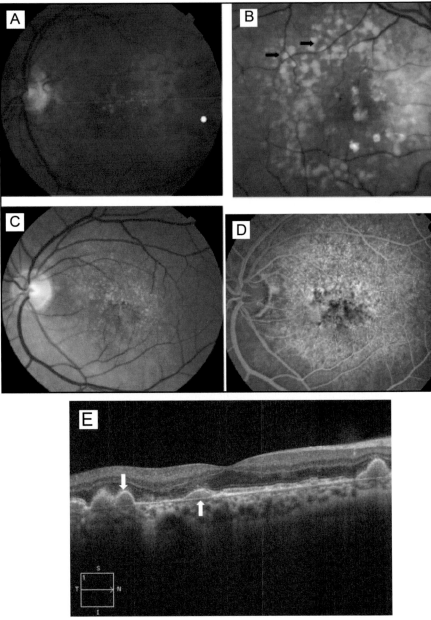

Figure 3-1. (A) Small, intermediate drusen in early-stage AMD. (B) Numerous large, soft drusen (arrows) and RPE changes in later-stage dry AMD. (C) Cuticular drusen. (D) Drusen appear more numerous on fluorescein angiography. (E) Optical coherence tomography scanning through drusen demonstrates excrescences at the level of Bruch's membrane.

vision, difficulty reading fine print, metamorphopsia, central or paracentral scotomata, color vision abnormalities, problems with glare and contrast, and poor dark adaptation.

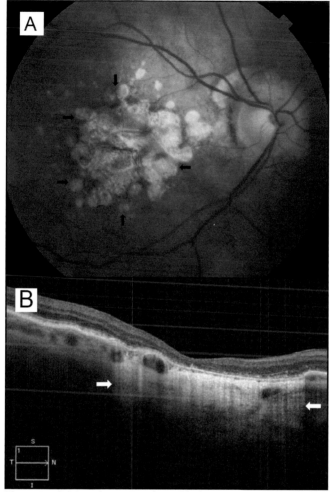

Figure 3-2. (A) Atrophic AMD with GA (black arrows). Note the choroidal vessels, which are visible under the area of atrophy. (B) Optical coherence tomography scanning through GA reveals retinal thinning, loss of outer retinal layers, and reverse shadowing (between arrows). Note the choroidal thinning, which is also characteristic.

Wet AMD usually presents unilaterally, with the sudden onset of metamorphopsia and/or decreased central vision.

SIGNS OF DRY AGE-RELATED MACULAR DEGENERATION

Drusen are yellowish deposits of extracellular debris located beneath the RPE. They are usually found in the macular region but may occur anywhere in the retina; however, the macular drusen contribute to a diagnosis of macular degeneration. The hallmarks of dry AMD are multiple small or any medium-sized or large drusen in the macula, with or without RPE abnormalities.[5,6] The diameter of drusen can be compared with the diameter of a normal retinal vein as it enters the optic nerve head, which is 125 µm in diameter, on average. Small drusen are < 63 µm, medium-sized drusen are ≥ 63 to < 125 µm, and large drusen are ≥ 125 µm in diameter.

Drusen can also be subclassified as hard or soft. Hard drusen are typically small, well-demarcated, yellow excrescences that may often be considered normal aging changes. However, the presence of numerous hard drusen is associated with an increased risk of progression to AMD. Soft drusen are larger and with more ill-defined borders; patients with soft drusen are almost always classified as having dry macular degeneration. Soft drusen may coalesce and form drusenoid pigment epithelial detachments. Soft drusen may also resolve spontaneously, which is sometimes accompanied by the development of RPE and choriocapillaris atrophy.

Basal laminar (cuticular) drusen are a variant of drusen that represent thickening of the basal membrane of the RPE. They are usually associated with a good visual prognosis and low risk of progression to wet macular degeneration. They appear on fluorescein angiography as numerous small, hyperfluorescent lesions (many more than are seen on clinical examination) and have a characteristic "starry sky" appearance.[7] Pseudovitelliform collections of yellowish subretinal material can occur in conjunction with basal laminar drusen.

Reticular pseudodrusen are seen as a reticular network of small, yellow lesions best seen using fundus autofluorescence (FAF) and/or blue-light fundus photography. Optical coherence tomography (OCT) shows that these lesions are located between the RPE and the retina, instead of underneath the RPE. These may be associated with an increased risk of progression to advanced stages of macular degeneration.[8]

Other changes that are characteristic of dry AMD include the presence of RPE hyper- or hypopigmentation and the presence of GA. Focal hyperpigmentation in the macula may be associated with an increased risk of the development of advanced AMD. Focal hypopigmentation may occur in isolation or in association with drusen. GA is a manifestation of the advanced form of dry AMD and is visualized as a well-demarcated area of RPE hypopigmentation, with visible underlying choroidal vasculature due to end stage RPE atrophy.[8,9]

SIGNS OF WET AGE-RELATED MACULAR DEGENERATION

Wet AMD is characterized by the presence of CNV, which may be sub-RPE or subretinal or, rarely, have intraretinal components. CNV may appear as a grayish or greenish subretinal membrane in the macular region. There may be associated intraretinal edema, RPE detachments, and/or subretinal fluid.[10] Associated lipid accumulations or hard exudates may be seen. Hemorrhages (sub-RPE, subretinal, intraretinal, or, rarely in the case of massive hemorrhage, preretinal or vitreous) may also be seen. Retinal pigment epithelial detachments may evolve into an RPE tear. The end stage of wet AMD is the development of a fibrous disciform scar, with resultant profound, irreversible visual loss.

SLIT-LAMP BIOMICROSCOPY

The diagnosis of dry AMD is primarily based on clinical examination of the macula, using a magnifying stereoscopic lens such as the 60-, 90-, or 78-diopter handheld lenses or, less commonly, a contact lens. In dry AMD, the presence and type of drusen, associated RPE changes, and GA can be directly visualized; these same changes can also be present in eyes that have CNV. In the wet form, serous elevation of the retina, macular hemorrhage, pigment epithelial detachments, intra- or subretinal fluid, hard exudates, and/or clinically visible subretinal CNV membranes are highly suggestive of the diagnosis of wet AMD, particularly in the setting of AMD changes in the fellow eye. However, ancillary imaging techniques, particularly fluorescein angiography (FA) and/or OCT, are usually needed to make or confirm the diagnosis.

RETINAL IMAGING

Chapter 4 discusses the following imaging techniques in greater detail. However, retinal imaging is discussed briefly here because it is often critical to the diagnosis and categorization of AMD.

Fluorescein Angiography

On FA, drusen typically appear as hyperfluorescent, well-circumscribed lesions that do not "leak."[6,11] GA appears as a well-demarcated "window defect." More important, FA is still believed to be the best method for the detection of new-onset CNV. The presence of CNV on FA can help to make or confirm the diagnosis of wet AMD and may be important in categorizing subtypes of wet AMD (Figure 3-3).

Optical Coherence Tomography

OCT has emerged as one of the most important tools in AMD. Not only is it useful in diagnosing early disease and documenting the extent of lesions, it is also critical in the management and assessment of response to treatment (Figure 3-4). It may be used in conjunction with other techniques to differentiate AMD from AMD mimickers. Serial OCTs are used to monitor the efficacy of treatment, determine disease activity, and examine microstructural changes in the retina, choroid, and vitreoretinal interface over time.[12-14]

Fundus Autofluorescence

FAF is an easy, quick, sensitive, and noninvasive tool that may aid in the diagnosis of AMD, particularly in measuring the area of GA or in differentiating AMD from AMD mimickers.[15]

Indocyanine Green Angiography

Indocyanine green angiography is generally less useful than FA in identifying CNV. However, it can be useful in differentiating wet AMD from potential masqueraders such as central serous chorioretinopathy and polypoidal choroidal vasculopathy and in identifying retinal angiomatous proliferation.[16]

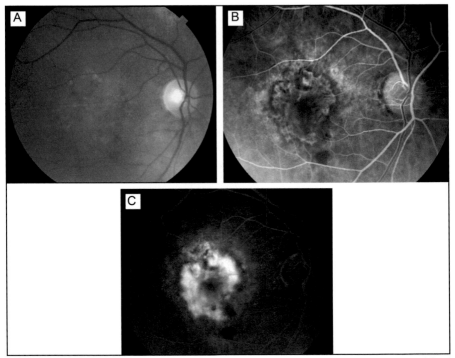

Figure 3-3. Classic choroidal neovascular membrane. (A) Color photograph shows subretinal fluid and hemorrhage. On fluorescein angiography, there is (B) early hyperfluorescence in a lacy pattern and (C) late leakage.

B-Scan Ultrasonography

In rare instances, when dense vitreous hemorrhage from the CNV precludes diagnosis or a large hemorrhagic macular lesion obscures a diagnosis, ocular ultrasonography provides useful information in the differentiation between CNV and choroidal tumors at the posterior pole due to different acoustic characteristics.[17]

CLASSIFICATION OF AGE-RELATED MACULAR DEGENERATION

Many different classification systems to describe AMD have been proposed. Most of these classifications have been developed to categorize the long-term risk of developing advanced disease and are based on findings from the Age-Related Eye Disease Study (AREDS).[18] In AREDS, patients were classified into 4 categories:

- *Category 1:* None or a few small drusen (< 63 μm)
- *Category 2:* Multiple small drusen, few intermediate drusen (63 to 124 μm), and/or retinal pigment epithelium abnormalities
- *Category 3:* Extensive intermediate drusen, at least one large drusen (≥ 125 μm), and/or GA not involving the fovea
- *Category 4:* GA involving the fovea and/or any of the features of wet AMD

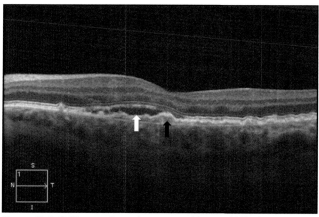

Figure 3-4. OCT scan through an eye with wet AMD demonstrates subretinal fluid (white arrow). Also note the underlying drusen (black arrow).

More recently, a committee of 26 AMD experts, 1 neuro-ophthalmologist, 2 committee chairmen, and 1 methodologist met to construct a more clear classification system of AMD.[19] This classification was based on assessment of the macula within a 2-disc-diameter radius of the center of the fovea and is as follows:

- *No apparent aging changes*: No drusen or RPE changes consistent with AMD.
- *Normal aging changes*: Small drusen (<63 µm) without pigmentary changes.
- *Early AMD*: Medium-sized drusen (≥63 to <125 µm) without pigmentary changes.
- *Intermediate AMD*: Medium-sized drusen with pigmentary abnormalities associated with AMD or any large drusen (≥125 µm).
- *Late AMD*: Any GA or CNV formation.

For wet AMD, an older but still widely used system was described by Gass,[20] who classified wet AMD into the subretinal and the sub-RPE types that corresponded with the classic and occult CNV membranes seen on FA. Later, Gass[20] used the terms *type 1* and *type 2*, and Freund et al[21] termed a third type of CNV:

- *Sub-RPE* (type 1): The CNV is confined to the sub-RPE space. This manifests on FA as an occult CNV.
- *Subretinal* (type 2): The CNV has gained access to the subretinal space through breaks in the RPE and grows in between the neurosensory retina and the RPE layer. This manifests on FA as a classic CNV.
- *Intraretinal* (type 3): Otherwise known as retinal angiomatous proliferation, type 3 CNV is intraretinal and was initially described by Freund et al.[21] This typically presents with intraretinal hemorrhage, exudates, and edema, in addition to other typical signs of CNV. In some cases, the anastomosis between the subretinal and intraretinal components is visible.

TABLE 3-1. AREDS ASSESSMENT OF RISK
FOR DEVELOPMENT OF ADVANCED DISEASE*

NO. OF RISK FACTORS	RISK, %
0	0.4
1	3.1
2	11.8
3	25.9
4	47.3

*One point per eye for the presence of large drusen; 1 point per eye for the presence of pigmentary changes; 1 point total for extensive intermediate drusen in both eyes; 2 points for advanced AMD in one eye.

Adapted from Ferris FL, Davis MD, Clemons TE, et al. A simplified severity scale for age-related macular degeneration: AREDS report no. 18. *Arch Ophthalmol.* 2005;123(11):1570-1574.

CLASSIFICATION BASED ON
FLUORESCEIN ANGIOGRAPHY APPEARANCE

A classification system based on FA findings was devised for wet AMD, which was especially relevant in the laser and photodynamic therapy era but is becoming less relevant in the era of anti-vascular endothelial growth factor (anti-VEGF) therapy.[11] On FA, CNV can be divided into 2 main types: classic CNV and occult CNV. The classification of wet AMD based on FA appearance is discussed in more detail in Chapter 4, Section 3.

Choroidal neovascular membranes that show combined features of classic and occult CNV are further subclassified into predominantly classic and minimally classic. Those that show classic features for at least 50% of their total area are called predominantly classic, whereas those that show classic features for less than 50% of their total area are called minimally classic.

Choroidal neovascular membranes can also be subdivided based on their relationship to the center of the foveal avascular zone (FAZ). CNV membranes are considered extrafoveal if they are ≥ 200 and < 2500 μm from the center of the FAZ, juxtafoveal if they are 1 to 199 μm from the center of the FAZ, and subfoveal if they involve the center of the FAZ.

RISK STRATIFICATION BASED ON
EXAMINATION FINDINGS

Using the original 4-category staging system used in the AREDS, the 5-year risk of developing advanced AMD in at least one eye was 1.3% for eyes in category 2, 18.3% in category 3, and 43.9% in category 4 (Table 3-1).[18] In 2005, the AREDS Research Group defined a "simplified severity scale" to help to better determine the risk of developing

TABLE 3-2. FIVE-YEAR RATES OF ADVANCED AMD (IN ONE OR BOTH EYES FOR PATIENTS WITH BOTH EYES AT RISK)

	PATIENTS WITHOUT ADVANCED AMD IN EITHER EYE AT BASELINE*			PATIENTS WITH ADVANCED AMD IN ONE EYE AT BASELINE†		
Risk Factors	No. at Risk	No. Who Developed Advanced AMD at 5 Years	%	No. at Risk	No. Who Developed Advanced AMD at 5 Years	%
0	1466	6	0.4			
1	635	20	3.1			
2	455	55	11.8	149	22	14.8
3	328	85	25.9	178	63	35.4
4	317	150	47.3	273	145	53.1

Abbreviation: AMD, age-related macular degeneration.

*Assign one risk factor for each eye with large drusen. Assign one risk factor for each eye with pigment abnormalities. Assign one risk factor if neither eye has large drusen and both eyes have intermediate drusen.

†Assign 2 risk factors for the eye that has neovascular AMD. Assign one additional risk factor if the eye at risk has large drusen. Assign one additional risk factor if the eye at risk has pigment abnormalities.

Reprinted with permission from Ferris FL, Davis MD, Clemons TE, et al. A simplified severity scale for age-related macular degeneration: AREDS report no. 18. *Arch Ophthalmol.* 2005;123(11):1570-1574.

advanced AMD based on clinical examination findings alone.[22] This scale was based on 3 observations: (1) the association of drusen size and drusen area with disease progression, (2) the low frequency of GA in the absence of RPE hyperpigmentation, and (3) the finding that large drusen in both eyes was a stronger risk factor for progression to advanced AMD than presence in only one eye. Based on these findings, the simplified severity scale was devised, and percentage of risk could be calculated and assigned to each severity level (Table 3-2). This risk stratification is derived from the clinical examination and is still used by clinicians to determine the 5-year prognosis, during discussions with patients, and in deciding the frequency of follow-up.

COUNSELING OF PATIENTS WITH AGE-RELATED MACULAR DEGENERATION

Treatment Regimens

Modifiable risk factors are discussed in more detail in Chapter 1. Patients diagnosed with AMD need to be counseled on lifestyle changes, dietary modifications (a diet high in carotenoids and lutein), smoking cessation, and weight management. Moreover, individuals with a diagnosis of intermediate or advanced macular degeneration should also be counseled on taking the modified AREDS2 multivitamin formula as a preventative treatment, unless otherwise contraindicated (see Chapter 1).[23] This includes the following components:

- 500 mg vitamin C
- 400 IU vitamin E
- 25 mg zinc oxide
- 2 mg cupric oxide
- 10 mg lutein and 2 mg zeaxanthin

Wet AMD management involves the addition of one or several types of active treatment. The first line of treatment is usually anti-VEGF therapy, but other forms of treatment, such as photodynamic therapy and focal laser, are also available. A discussion of the risks and benefits of the recommended treatment or treatments should occur with each patient so that he or she can provide informed consent and help to choose the treatment course that best suits him or her. Treatment methods for wet AMD are discussed in detail later in this book.

Home Monitoring

Monocular home testing is important for the early detection of new changes because conversion to wet AMD may cause rapid disease progression and irreversible damage to vision, which may go unnoticed by the patient if he or she compensates with the fellow eye. The Amsler grid has long been considered an important and easy self-assessment tool used to monitor the status of central vision (central 20 degrees of the visual field around fixation) in AMD patients and to detect new central or paracentral scotomata and metamorphopsia. Patients are given an Amsler grid to check monocular central vision regularly, at least on a weekly basis, and should seek urgent ophthalmologist consultation if new changes appear.

However, the classic Amsler grid is not able to provide quantitative results. A computerized Amsler grid has also been generated for AMD patients and may have better sensitivity in screening for both forms of AMD, assessing disease severity, differentiating between atrophic and exudative AMD, and providing quantitative measurements of response to therapy.[24,25] Many other home testing aids have also been devised and may have additional advantages for the self-monitoring of patients considered to be at high risk. These may be more sensitive in diagnosing new scotomata due to the development of CNV. These aids include preferential hyperacuity perimetry (ForeseeHome; Notal Vision Ltd), the macular mapping test, and the noise-field campimeter, among others.[26-29] However, none of these tests are currently commonly used in clinical practice.

Low Vision

Finally, patients with vision loss due to advanced AMD may benefit from visual rehabilitative/low-vision services that enable them to maximize the use of the vision they have. This may include training to optimize lighting, using high contrast and large print, magnification lenses for reading, strategies to mitigate the visual effects of blind spots, and visual aids, such as closed-circuit television for patients with more severe vision loss.

SUMMARY

Patients are routinely diagnosed with AMD based on typical symptoms and signs on fundus biomicroscopy. AMD may be classified as dry (atrophic, non-neovascular) or wet (exudative, neovascular). Certain characteristics on examination, as well as ancillary testing, aid in the diagnosis of AMD. Characteristics such as larger-sized drusen, pigmentary abnormalities, and advanced AMD in the fellow eye are associated with a higher risk of progression of AMD. Patients with intermediate or advanced AMD are counseled to take vitamin supplements as directed by AREDS2. Patients with AMD are also counseled to monitor vision at home using the Amsler grid or other home monitoring devices. Low-vision evaluation and counseling may be recommended for patients with advanced forms of AMD.

REFERENCES

1. Klein R, Klein BEK, Jensen SC, Meuer SM. The five-year incidence and progression of age-related maculopathy. The Beaver Dam Eye Study. *Ophthalmology.* 1997;104:7-21.

2. Bressler NM, Munoz B, Maguire MG, et al. Five-year incidence and disappearance of drusen and retinal pigment epithelial abnormalities. Waterman Study. *Arch Ophthalmol.* 1995;113:301-308.

3. Lee MY, Yoon J, Ham DI. Clinical features of reticular pseudodrusen according to fundus distribution. *Br J Ophthalmol.* 2012;96(9):1222-1226.

4. Bressler NM, Silva JC, Bressler SB, Fine SL, Green WR. Clinicopathologic correlation of drusen and retinal pigment epithelial abnormalities in age-related macular degeneration. *Retina.* 1994;14(2):130-142.

5. Abdelsalam A, Del Priore L, Zarbin MA. Drusen in age-related macular degeneration: pathogenesis, natural course, and laser photocoagulation-induced regression. *Surv Ophthalmol.* 1999;44(1):1-29.

6. Spaide RF, Curcio CA. Drusen characterization with multimodal imaging. *Retina.* 2010;30(9):1441-1454.

7. Russell SR, Mullins RF, Schneider BL, Hageman GS. Location, substructure, and composition of basal laminar drusen compared with drusen associated with aging and age-related macular degeneration. *Am J Ophthalmol.* 2000;129(2):205-214.

8. Zweifel SA, Imamura Y, Spaide TC, Fujiwara T, Spaide RF. Prevalence and significance of subretinal drusenoid deposits (reticular pseudodrusen) in age-related macular degeneration. *Ophthalmology.* 2010;117(9):1775-1781.

9. Bird AC, Bressler NM, Bressler SB, et al. An international classification and grading system for age-related maculopathy and age-related macular degeneration. The International ARM Epidemiological Study Group. *Surv Ophthalmol.* 1995;39(5):367-374.

10. Biarnés M, Monés J, Alonso J, Arias L. Update on geographic atrophy in age-related macular degeneration. *Optom Vis Sci.* 2011;88(7):881-889.

11. Barbezetto I, Burdan A, Bressler NM, et al. Photodynamic therapy of subfoveal choroidal neovascularization with verteporfin: fluorescein angiographic guidelines for evaluation and treatment— TAP and VIP report No. 2. *Arch Ophthalmol.* 2003;121(9):1253-1268.

12. Tan CS, Heussen F, Sadda SR. Peripheral autofluorescence and clinical findings in neovascular and non-neovascular age-related macular degeneration. *Ophthalmology*. 2013;120(6):1271-1277.

13. Lumbroso B, Rispoli M. *Practical Handbook of OCT: Retina, Choroid, Glaucoma*. New Dehli, India: Jaypee Brothers Medical Publishers; 2012.

14. Adhi M, Duker JS. Optical coherence tomography—current and future applications. *Curr Opin Ophthalmol*. 2013;24(3):213-221.

15. Cuba JJ, Gómez-Ulla F. Fundus autofluorescence: applications and perspectives. *Arch Soc Esp Oftalmol*. 2013;88(2):50-55.

16. Fernandes LH, Freund KB, Yannuzzi LA, et al. The nature of focal areas of hyperfluorescence or hot spots imaged with indocyanine green angiography. *Retina*. 2002;22:557-568.

17. Kubicka-Trzaska A. Differential diagnosis of exudative age-related macular degeneration with posterior pole choroidal tumors [in German]. *Klin Oczna*. 2005;107(1-3):147-155.

18. Age-Related Eye Disease Study Research Group. A randomized, placebo-controlled, clinical trial of high-dose supplementation with vitamins C and E, beta carotene, and zinc for age-related macular degeneration and vision loss: AREDS report no. 8. *Arch Ophthalmol*. 2001;119(10):1417-1436.

19. Ferris FL III, Wilkinson CP, Bird A, et al. Clinical classification of age-related macular degeneration. *Ophthalmology*. 2013;120(4):844-851.

20. Gass JDM. Biomicroscopic and histologic considerations regarding the feasibility of surgical excision of subfoveal neovascular membranes. *Am J Ophthalmol*. 1994;18:285-298.

21. Freund KB, Ho IV, Barbazetto IA, et al. Type 3 neovascularization: the expanded spectrum of retinal angiomatous proliferation. *Retina*. 2008;28(2):201-211.

22. Ferris FL, Davis MD, Clemons TE, et al. A simplified severity scale for age-related macular degeneration: AREDS Report No. 18. *Arch Ophthalmol*. 2005;123(11):1570-1574.

23. Age-Related Eye Disease Study 2 Research Group. Lutein + zeaxanthin and omega-3 fatty acids for age-related macular degeneration: the Age-Related Eye Disease Study 2 (AREDS2) randomized clinical trial. *JAMA*. 2013;309(19):2005-2015.

24. Frisén L. The Amsler grid in modern clothes. *Br J Ophthalmol*. 2009;93(6):714-716.

25. Robison CD, Jivrajka RV, Bababeygy SR, Fink W, Sadun AA, Sebag J. Distinguishing wet from dry age-related macular degeneration using three-dimensional computer-automated threshold Amsler grid testing. *Br J Ophthalmol*. 2011;95(10):1419-1423.

26. Trevino R. Recent progress in macular function self-assessment. *Ophthalmic Physiol Opt*. 2008;28(3):183-192.

27. Do DV. Detection of new-onset choroidal neovascularization. *Curr Opin Ophthalmol*. 2013;24(3):244-247.

28. Meyer CH, Lapolice DJ. Computer-based visual evaluation as a screening tool after intravitreal injections of vascular endothelial growth factor inhibitors. *Ophthalmologica*. 2008;222(6):364-368.

29. The AREDS2-HOME Study Research Group, Chew WC, Clemons TE, et al. Randomized trial of a home monitoring system for early detection of choroidal neovascularization home monitoring of the eye (HOME) Study. *Ophthalmology*. 2014;121(2):535-544.

4

Ancillary Testing in Age-Related Macular Degeneration

Section 1: Fundus Photography and Autofluorescence

S.K. Steven Houston III, MD and Sunir J. Garg, MD, FACS

Paralleling the advances in age-related macular degeneration (AMD) treatment are advancements in retinal imaging, including color fundus photography and fundus autofluorescence (FAF).

BASICS OF FUNDUS PHOTOGRAPHY AND FUNDUS AUTOFLUORESCENCE

Fundus photographs help document the presence or absence of pathology, aid in monitoring disease progression, and act as a valuable educational tool for both physicians and patients. Traditionally, fundus photography has been performed using film, but in the past decade, most clinicians have adopted digital fundus photography. Digital images enable easy and immediate review, straightforward image magnification, and comparison of prior images. In AMD, color fundus photography is often obtained at baseline to enable clinical comparisons over time and to document new findings. In addition, fundus photography currently serves as the gold standard to grade dry AMD in clinical research studies.

By exciting fluorophores in the fundus and then using subsequent filters to capture the emission from these fluorophores, FAF noninvasively highlights natural and pathologic changes affecting the retinal pigment epithelium (RPE) (Figure 4-1-1). The primary fluorophore of the retina is lipofuscin, a byproduct of photoreceptor outer-segment accumulation.[1] The main fluorophore constituent of lipofuscin is A2E, a bisretinoid involved in the visual cycle.[2] Accumulation of these by-products not only interferes with normal RPE cellular function but is also toxic to the RPE.[3] FAF imaging can be obtained with confocal scanning laser ophthalmoscopy or a modified fundus camera. Excitation light wavelengths for confocal scanning laser ophthalmoscopy are

Witkin AJ, Duker JS, eds.
*Age-Related Macular Degeneration:
Current Management (pp. 43-74)*
© 2015 Taylor & Francis Group

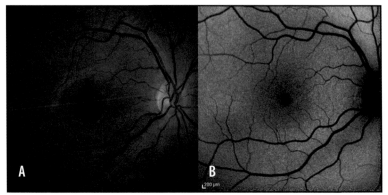

Figure 4-1-1. (A) Normal color fundus photograph and (B) FAF of the right eye.

approximately 480 nm, whereas modified fundus cameras use slightly longer wavelengths, approximately 532 nm. Emission filters for confocal scanning laser ophthalmoscopy range from 500 to 700 nm, whereas those of fundus cameras range from 600 to 700 nm. FAF of normal eyes shows a characteristic pattern. Blood vessels and the optic nerve are hypoautofluorescent (hypoAF), whereas the fovea shows variable hypoAF secondary to absorption of light by lutein and zeaxanthin at the excitation wavelength. Pathologic FAF patterns in AMD can be hyperautofluorescent (hyperAF) or hypoAF, with specific patterns possibly serving as a predictor of progression.

EARLY TO INTERMEDIATE AMD: DRUSEN

Fundus photography of eyes with early AMD demonstrates a number of findings, but drusenoid changes are the hallmark features. Drusen can be divided into hard and soft types. They vary in size and distribution and may have sharp (discrete) or soft (indiscrete) borders. Drusen size can be measured by comparing the width of an ophthalmic vein at the disc margin, which is approximately 125 µm in diameter. Small drusen are defined as those equal to or less than 63 µm (or half of the size of the vein diameter); large drusen are greater than 125 µm in size. Intermediate drusen are those that are sized between small and large, measuring 64 to 125 µm (Figures 4-1-2 and 4-1-3). This classification enables standardized grading of AMD, which is important for risk stratifying patients (see Chapter 3).

FAF of early AMD demonstrates a variety of different patterns and changes, reflecting activity at the level of the RPE. Medium to large drusen typically have a central area of hypoAF with an outer ring of hyperAF.[4] Smaller drusen may not show any notable changes on FAF, and larger drusen may be more heterogenous in appearance. There is debate as to what actually causes the drusen appearance on FAF, including loss of the RPE cells, peripheral displacement of the RPE cells by the underlying druse, and increased AF due to vertically superimposed cells and cellular fragments rather than from lipofuscin.[5] In addition, FAF can demonstrate RPE abnormalities that are not visible through fundus photographs. Some investigators suggest that FAF changes may represent changes to RPE health and serve as a predictor of AMD progression.[6]

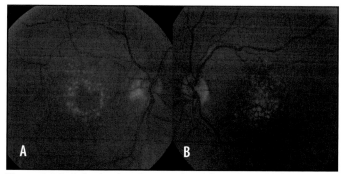

Figure 4-1-2. Color fundus photographs of the right and left eyes show (A) small, intermediate, and large drusen and (B) small and intermediate drusen.

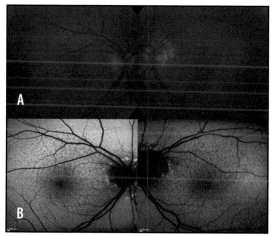

Figure 4-1-3. (A) Color fundus photographs of the right and left eyes show small to intermediate drusen. (B) FAF shows hypoAF corresponding to the drusen.

Bindewald et al[7] developed a classification system of early AMD based on FAF findings. The classification includes 1 normal pattern and 7 abnormal patterns that are seen in eyes with dry AMD: minimal change, focal increased, patchy, linear, lace-like, reticular, and speckled. This classification varies considerably from standard fundus photographic changes, suggesting that FAF changes may identify different phenotypes along this disease spectrum. The minimal change pattern displays a few irregular hypoAF or hyperAF areas. Focal increased displays focal hyperAF less than 200 μm in diameter that do not necessarily correlate with fundoscopic changes. Patchy patterns are similar to the focal increased pattern but are 200 μm or larger and have less well-defined borders. Linear patterns display areas of linear hyperAF that correspond to hyperpigmented areas on fundoscopy. Lace-like patterns display more advanced linear patterns with branching. Finally, reticular patterns display an overall background AF with areas of small hypoAF less than 200 μm in diameter. Reticular patterns have been associated with advanced disease, GA, and choroidal neovascularization (CNV) and have been shown to be as high as 36% in the contralateral eyes of patients with CNV.[8] In a study of 458 patients with GA, 62% were found to have a reticular pattern on FAF.[9] Reticular patterns have also been shown to enlarge over time, but this rate of enlargement has not been correlated with rates of progression to advanced disease.[10] Future studies need to correlate specific FAF patterns with AMD genetic profiles, the risk for progression to advanced disease, and its use in identifying high-risk patients for clinical trials of therapeutic treatments for dry AMD.

RETINAL PIGMENT EPITHELIAL DETACHMENT

Retinal pigment epithelial detachments (RPEDs) can be seen in a number of diseases and are common in patients with AMD. RPEDs occur in both dry and wet AMD and present as dome-shaped elevations. RPEDs may be drusenoid, serous, vascular, or mixed. RPEDs are often associated with an underlying CNV. Although the presence of blood, overlying subretinal fluid, or lipid exudation is a clue to an exudative process, it is often difficult to determine the type of RPED based on fundus examination alone. Although fluorescein angiography (FA) and optical coherence tomography (OCT) are critical to determine the presence of underlying CNV, color photographs and FAF can be helpful as well.

Drusenoid RPEDs are a form of dry AMD. On color photographs, they appear as yellowish elevations that often have overlying pigmentary changes. Serous RPEDs appear as clear, sharply demarcated, dome-shaped elevations that have an increased risk for CNV development. Patients with AMD and serous RPEDs have a 28% to 39% incidence of developing a CNV over the next 2 years.[11-14] Fibrovascular RPEDs appear either as regular elevations that look similar to serous RPEDs or as irregular elevations that may be associated with other features, such as blood, edema exudation, or chorioretinal folds. Gass[15] reported that a flattened border or notch is commonly seen in RPEDs associated with a CNV.

RPEDs may have varying appearances on FAF images but are typically isoautofluorescent (isoAF) or hyperAF, with a ring of hypoAF delineating the boundary of the RPEDs.[16,17] RPEDs with overlying pigment or RPE changes may also show some degree of focal hyperAF. The source of autofluorescent signal from RPEDs is a matter of debate and includes lipofuscin, undetermined fluorophores, serous fluid, and degraded photoreceptors.[18] Not much work has been done to identify patterns on FAF that may help identify ibrovascular RPEDs from serous or drusenoid RPEDs. OCT and FA are still the gold standards in these cases.

GEOGRAPHIC ATROPHY

GA represents an advanced form of dry AMD associated with RPE loss and atrophy that affects the overlying photoreceptors. GA can result in vision loss that can be as severe as that of advanced wet AMD. The exact mechanisms for GA are not completely known. Currently, there are no treatments to restore vision loss from GA, but various medications and stem cell therapies are in early clinical trials to investigate their safety and efficacy in GA.

Fundus photographs of GA show areas of depigmentation or RPE loss of 175 μm or more in size, with increased visibility of underlying choroidal vessels.[19] FAF of GA shows distinct hypoAF areas corresponding to the areas of RPE loss (Figures 4-1-4 and 4-1-5). FAF often demonstrates more extensive areas than may be seen by fundus photography or clinical

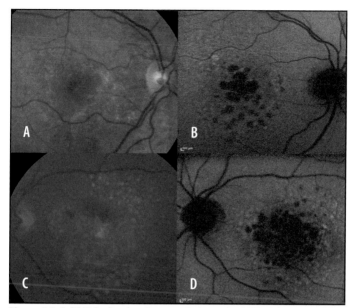

Figure 4-1-4. (A) Color fundus photograph shows dry AMD with scattered drusen and central GA. (B) FAF better delineates areas and borders of GA (hypoAF). (C) Color fundus photograph demonstrates an eye with extensive GA with exudation along the superior portion of the area of atrophy. (D) FAF demonstrates the areas of GA (hypoAF).

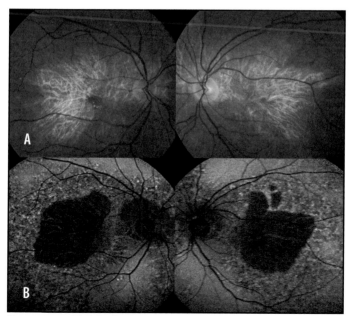

Figure 4-1-5. (A) Color fundus photographs show GA, with visualization of underlying choroidal vessels. (B) FAF shows hypofluorescent GA with diffuse, trickling junctional zone pattern. This autofluorescence pattern has a high rate of GA progression.

TABLE 4-1-1. GEOGRAPHIC ATROPHY ENLARGEMENT OVER TIME

FAF PATTERN	GA GROWTH RATE, MM^2 PER YEAR
None	0.38
Focal	0.81
Diffuse (nontrickling)	1.67
Banded	1.81
Diffuse trickling	3.02

Adapted from Holz FG, Bindewald-Wittich A, Fleckenstein M, Dreyhaupt J, Scholl HP, Schmitz-Valckenberg S. Progression of geographic atrophy and impact of fundus autofluorescence patterns in age-related macular degeneration. *Am J Ophthalmol.* 2007;143:463-472.

examination. The junctional zone between the otherwise healthy-appearing retina and the areas of atrophy has stimulated significant interest. The junctional zone often exhibits hyperAF and has been associated with both increased growth of atrophic areas and the development of new atrophy.[6] There is also remarkable symmetry between a patient's eyes, with up to 80% demonstrating similar GA patterns[20] and rates of progression, but there is often asymmetry in GA size.[21]

Investigators conducted the Fundus Autofluorescence Imaging in Age-Related Macular Degeneration (FAM) study to evaluate the natural history of GA progression. Based on FAF patterns at the junctional zone, the FAM study investigators proposed a classification system to correlate the risk of GA progression with FAF appearance.[22] In this prospective longitudinal study, 195 eyes with GA were followed over a median of 1.8 years. The investigators found a wide range of GA progression, from 0.38 mm^2 per year to 3.02 mm^2 per year, with a mean of 1.74 mm^2 per year. GA patterns were based on hyperAF of the junctional zone. Initial classification included (1) none, which is no area of increased junctional FAF; (2) diffuse, which is diffuse FAF at the margins; and (3) FAF at the margins and elsewhere in the posterior pole. For diffuse FAF, subtypes included reticular, branching, fine granular, fine granular with peripheral punctuate spots, and trickling. For patients with FAF at the margins, subtypes included focal, banded, and patchy. Analysis showed that none and focal patterns showed the slowest rates of progression, whereas the banded and diffuse patterns showed the highest rates of progression. Within the diffuse classification, trickling had the highest rate of progression (3.02 mm^2 per year) among all FAF patterns (Table 4-1-1).[22] The Geographic Atrophy Progression (GAP) study evaluated the distribution and progression of GA in 413 eyes.[23] Those investigators found that foveal and parafoveal areas, as well as areas superior to the macula, were more prone to GA and progression. These studies suggested that different phenotypes within the GA spectrum behave differently and warrant further evaluation and study. These findings also need further correlation with visual outcomes. FAF characteristics may serve as useful outcome measures for clinical trials and identifying high-risk individuals for clinical interventions.

FAF studies have hypothesized that junctional-zone hyperAF occurs secondary to the accumulation of lipofuscin and that these areas are more prone to RPE cell death with

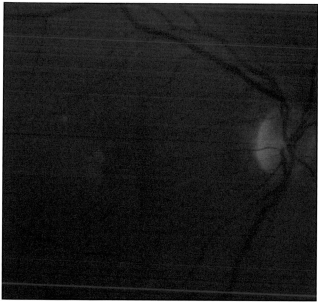

Figure 4-1-6. Right eye with scattered small and intermediate drusen, as well as a juxtafoveal grayish elevation corresponding to a CNV.

atrophy progression. Other studies have shown that atrophy progression does not necessarily progress at local areas of hyperAF,[24] but overall patterns of hyperAF contribute to risk of progression.[22] Histopathologic autofluorescence studies have shown RPE alterations at the border of atrophic areas, including cellular rounding, sloughing, and layering.[5] Of note, peaks in intensity of histopathologic autofluorescence adjacent to atrophic areas often resulted from vertically superimposed cells and cellular fragments, rather than from lipofuscin alone. As a result, increased FAF may highlight areas of advanced RPE morphologic changes and alterations[5] but may not necessarily highlight diseased RPE cells on the verge of death. These studies emphasize the importance of continued investigation of disease mechanisms for GA and that lipofuscin toxicity may not be the final step in the disease pathway.

CHOROIDAL NEOVASCULARIZATION

CNV represents the defining characteristic of wet AMD. Type 1 CNV occurs under the RPE, type 2 occurs above the RPE,[25] and type 3 is distinguished by retinochoroidal anastomosis.[26] Wet AMD is the leading cause of blindness in the developed world in patients aged 55 years and older. With the advent of anti-vascular endothelial growth factor (anti-VEGF) treatment, loss of 15 or more letters can be prevented in more than 90% of patients, with more than 30% of patients gaining 15 or more letters.[27]

Fundus photographs of CNV may show a grayish-green subretinal elevation, although some patients may have only subtle subretinal elevation (Figure 4-1-6). The presence of subretinal fluid, blood, exudation, or RPE folds are important clinical findings often associated with CNV. CNV may also present as an RPED, with sharp demarcation of its borders. FA and OCT are important tools to confirm the diagnosis. FAF imaging in wet

AMD demonstrates a myriad of patterns, depending on the overlying RPE disruption. FAF may remain normal in early-stage CNV.[28] Lipid, blood, and subretinal fibrosis cause hypoAF. HyperAF may be found inferiorly from guttering of fluid.

Studies assessing differences in FAF for occult and classic CNVs have shown mixed results.[28,29] FAF has been investigated as a predictor for anti-VEGF response, also with mixed and inconclusive results.[30,31] Finally, in the FAM study, 9 (7.2%) of 125 eyes developed CNV. Six (67%) of 9 patients who developed CNV had a patchy FAF pattern. FAF for the other 3 patients included both focal and reticular patterns.[32] FAF patterns in patients with wet AMD and those at high risk of developing CNV have not been studied at length. Further studies are needed to determine the ability of FAF to predict eyes that may develop wet AMD.

SUMMARY

Color fundus photography and FAF are valuable tools in an ophthalmologists' armamentarium. Fundus photography documents baseline findings and makes following patients with both dry and wet AMD easier over time. FAF has also emerged as a useful imaging modality, especially in patients with dry AMD. Despite a lack of therapeutic options for vision loss from dry AMD, FAF provides detailed information regarding GA size, progression, and patterns predictive of disease progression. FAF appears to be most useful to follow patients with GA over time and to serve as an outcome measure to evaluate experimental therapies. Color fundus photography and FAF will continue to complement other imaging modalities in the diagnosis and management of patients with AMD.

REFERENCES

1. Feeney-Burns L, Berman ER, Rothman H. Lipofuscin of human retinal pigment epithelium. *Am J Ophthalmol*. 1980;90:783-791.
2. Sparrow JR, Kim SR, Wu Y. Experimental approaches to the study of A2E, a bisretinoid lipofuscin chromophore of retinal pigment epithelium. *Methods Mol Biol*. 2010;652:315-327.
3. Schutt F, Davies S, Kopitz J, Holz FG, Boulton ME. Photodamage to human RPE cells by A2-E, a retinoid component of lipofuscin. *Invest Ophthalmol Vis Sci*. 2000;41:2303-2308.
4. Delori FC, Fleckner MR, Goger DG, Weiter JJ, Dorey CK. Autofluorescence distribution associated with drusen in age-related macular degeneration. *Invest Ophthalmol Vis Sci*. 2000;41:496-504.
5. Rudolf M, Vogt SD, Curcio CA, et al. Histologic basis of variations in retinal pigment epithelium autofluorescence in eyes with geographic atrophy. *Ophthalmology*. 2013;120:821-828.
6. Holz FG, Bellman C, Staudt S, Schutt F, Volcker HE. Fundus autofluorescence and development of geographic atrophy in age-related macular degeneration. *Invest Ophthalmol Vis Sci*. 2001;42:1051-1056.
7. Bindewald A, Bird AC, Dandekar SS, et al. Classification of fundus autofluorescence patterns in early age-related macular disease. *Invest Ophthalmol Vis Sci*. 2005;46:3309-3314.
8. Smith RT, Chan JK, Busuoic M, Sivagnanavel V, Bird AC, Chong NV. Autofluorescence characteristics of early, atrophic, and high-risk fellow eyes in age-related macular degeneration. *Invest Ophthalmol Vis Sci*. 2006;47:5495-5504.
9. Schmitz-Valckenberg S, Alten F, Steinberg JS, et al. Reticular drusen associated with geographic atrophy in age-related macular degeneration. *Invest Ophthalmol Vis Sci*. 2011;52:5009-5015.
10. Steinberg JS, Auge J, Jaffe GJ, Fleckenstein M, Holz FG, Schmitz-Valckenberg S. Longitudinal analysis of reticular drusen associated with geographic atrophy in age-related macular degeneration. *Invest Ophthalmol Vis Sci*. 2013;54:4054-4060.

11. Elman MJ, Fine SL, Murphy RP, Patz A, Auer C. The natural history of serous retinal pigment epithelium detachment in patients with age-related macular degeneration. *Ophthalmology.* 1986;93:224-230.

12. Hartnett ME, Weiter JJ, Garsd A, Jalkh AE. Classification of retinal pigment epithelial detachments associated with drusen. *Graefes Arch Clin Exp Ophthalmol.* 1992;230:11-19.

13. Meredith TA, Braley RE, Aaberg TM. Natural history of serous detachments of the retinal pigment epithelium. *Am J Ophthalmol.* 1979;88:643-651.

14. Poliner LS, Olk RJ, Burgess D, Gordon ME. Natural history of retinal pigment epithelial detachments in age-related macular degeneration. *Ophthalmology.* 1986;93:543-551.

15. Gass JD. Serous retinal pigment epithelial detachment with a notch: a sign of occult choroidal neovascularization. *Retina.* 1984;4:205-220.

16. Schmitz-Valckenberg S, Fleckenstein M, Scholl HP, Holz FG. Fundus autofluorescence and progression of age-related macular degeneration. *Surv Ophthalmol.* 2009;54:96-117.

17. Karadimas P, Bouzas EA. Fundus autofluorescence imaging in serous and drusenoid pigment epithelial detachments associated with age-related macular degeneration. *Am J Ophthalmol.* 2005;140:1163-1165.

18. Roth F, Holz FG. Age-related macular degeneration III: pigment epithelium detachment. In: Holz F, Spaide R, Bird AC, Schmitz-Valckenberg S, eds. *Atlas of Fundus Autofluorescence Imaging.* Heidelberg, Germany: Springer; 2007:165-178.

19. Bird AC, Bressler NM, Bressler SB, et al. An international classification and grading system for age-related maculopathy and age-related macular degeneration. The International ARM Epidemiological Study Group. *Surv Ophthalmol.* 1995;39:367-374.

20. Bellmann C, Jorzik J, Spital G, Unnebrink K, Pauleikhoff D, Holz FG. Symmetry of bilateral lesions in geographic atrophy in patients with age-related macular degeneration. *Arch Ophthalmol.* 2002;120:579-584.

21. Fleckenstein M, Adrion C, Schmitz-Valckenberg S, et al. Concordance of disease progression in bilateral geographic atrophy due to AMD. *Invest Ophthalmol Vis Sci.* 2010;51:637-642.

22. Holz FG, Bindewald-Wittich A, Fleckenstein M, Dreyhaupt J, Scholl HP, Schmitz-Valckenberg S. Progression of geographic atrophy and impact of fundus autofluorescence patterns in age-related macular degeneration. *Am J Ophthalmol.* 2007;143:463-472.

23. Mauschitz MM, Fonseca S, Chang P, et al. Topography of geographic atrophy in age-related macular degeneration. *Invest Ophthalmol Vis Sci.* 2012;53:4932-4939.

24. Hwang JC, Chan JW, Chang S, Smith RT. Predictive value of fundus autofluorescence for development of geographic atrophy in age-related macular degeneration. *Invest Ophthalmol Vis Sci.* 2006;47:2655-2661.

25. Gass JD. Biomicroscopic and histopathologic considerations regarding the feasibility of surgical excision of subfoveal neovascular membranes. *Am J Ophthalmol.* 1994;118:285-298.

26. Freund KB, Ho IV, Barbazetto IA, et al. Type 3 neovascularization: the expanded spectrum of retinal angiomatous proliferation. *Retina.* 2008;28:201-211.

27. Rosenfeld PJ, Brown DM, Heier JS, et al. Ranibizumab for neovascular age-related macular degeneration. *N Engl J Med.* 2006;355:1419-1431.

28. Vaclavik V, Vujosevic S, Dandekar SS, Bunce C, Peto T, Bird AC. Autofluorescence imaging in age-related macular degeneration complicated by choroidal neovascularization: a prospective study. *Ophthalmology.* 2008;115:342-346.

29. McBain VA, Townend J, Lois N. Fundus autofluorescence in exudative age-related macular degeneration. *Br J Ophthalmol.* 2007;91:491-496.

30. Heimes B, Lommatzsch A, Zeimer M, et al. Foveal RPE autofluorescence as a prognostic factor for anti-VEGF therapy in exudative AMD. *Graefes Arch Clin Exp Ophthalmol.* 2008;246:1229-1234.

31. Chhablani J, Kozak IR, Mojana F, et al. Fundus autofluorescence not predictive of treatment response to intravitreal bevacizumab in exudative age-related macular degeneration. *Retina.* 2012;32:1465-1470.

32. Einbock W, Moessner A, Schnurrbusch UE, Holz FG, Wolf S. Changes in fundus autofluorescence in patients with age-related maculopathy. Correlation to visual function: a prospective study. *Graefes Arch Clin Exp Ophthalmol.* 2005;243:300-305.

4

SECTION 2: OPTICAL COHERENCE TOMOGRAPHY

Andre J. Witkin, MD

Optical coherence tomography (OCT) is an imaging technique capable of evaluating retinal morphology with microscopic resolution, essentially capturing an in vivo "optical biopsy."[1] Since it became commercially available in 1996, a steady progression of software and hardware improvements to OCT instruments occurred, and with the introduction of the Stratus OCT (Carl Zeiss Meditec, Dublin, California) in 2002, the technology emerged as an integral piece in the diagnosis and management of a variety of macular diseases. With the advent of anti-vascular endothelial growth factor (anti-VEGF) therapies for age-related macular degeneration (AMD) in 2006, the position of OCT as the most important ancillary test in AMD management and clinical decision making became clear.[2]

HOW OPTICAL COHERENCE TOMOGRAPHY WORKS

Similar to the way sound is used in ultrasound to create an image of tissue, OCT works by emitting light and then measuring the resultant echo time delay, or the time it takes for light to be reflected back from the target tissue. By rapidly scanning the OCT light source across the macula, multiple OCT A-scans may be obtained and combined to form a linear image analogous to a B-scan ultrasound image. Because light travels too fast to be detected directly, the echo time delay must be measured indirectly using a technique called low coherence interferometry.[1,3]

In OCT, the axial resolution is determined by the bandwidth of the light source. Older generations of OCT instruments (time-domain [TD]-OCT) used light sources capable of 10-µm axial resolution in the human eye. Recently, wider bandwidth light sources have been used that improve the ability to localize echoes within a target, thereby increasing axial resolution. Axial resolution in current spectral-domain (SD)-OCT devices ranges from 3 to 7 µm. Transverse resolution is independent of the bandwidth of the light and is dependent on the optical focusing of light on the retina. Transverse resolution in commercially available OCT instruments is limited to 10 to 15 µm by natural aberrations in the human eye.[4]

In older OCT systems (TD-OCT), a reference mirror was continuously moved to detect the OCT signal at varying depths within tissue. In SD-OCT devices, the OCT signal is detected using a stationary reference arm, allowing faster imaging speeds than in TD-OCT systems, and a greater wealth of OCT data becomes obtainable in an even shorter scan time.[5] SD-OCT systems are widely available commercially and have allowed even more detailed analysis of macular microstructures in healthy and diseased eyes.

Analysis software is critical to the function of OCT devices. Computer algorithms are used to calculate retinal thickness by automatically delineating the inner and outer retinal boundaries. When several OCT images are obtained through the macula, a map of retinal thickness can be generated. Previous TD-OCT systems acquired 6 linear images centered at the point of fixation, spaced 30 degrees apart, and typically 6 mm in length. Newer SD-OCT systems create macular maps using a much larger amount of OCT data. Images in SD-OCT systems are typically taken in a raster series to create macular thickness maps. Automated measurements of retinal thickness can then be compared with normative databases and followed over time (Figure 4-2-1).[2]

ENHANCED-DEPTH IMAGING

In SD-OCT, resolution and sensitivity decline as the distance of the target tissue increases from the top of the SD-OCT image (the zero-delay line). Typically, when an OCT image is acquired, the vitreoretinal interface is placed near the zero-delay line by the OCT technician, whereas the poorest OCT signal and resolution are in the outer retina and choroid. To enhance signal and resolution within the choroid using SD-OCT, the OCT instrument can be pushed closer to the eye to obtain an inverted image. This inverted image places the outer retina and choroid near the zero-delay line, increasing visualization of deep retinal and choroidal structures. Further enhancement of the signal can be obtained by image averaging, or averaging a number of identical B-scans to enhance the signal-to-noise ratio. The combination of these techniques is called enhanced-depth imaging OCT (EDI-OCT).[6] With EDI-OCT, it is possible to image the outer retina and choroid in greater detail. EDI-OCT may add additional information to the diagnosis and analysis of AMD.

OPTICAL COHERENCE TOMOGRAPHY IN HEALTHY EYES

OCT measures changes in optical reflectivity in the retina. Although these optical reflections are not identical to retinal structures, a high correlation between OCT and retinal histology has been shown.[7] Nerve fiber layers (retinal nerve fiber layer and inner and outer plexiform layers) are more highly reflective on OCT, whereas cell body layers (ganglion cell layer and inner and outer nuclear layers) are less highly reflective. The outer aspect of the neurosensory retina contains 4 closely spaced reflective layers. The innermost layer is less reflective and is thought to represent the external limiting membrane. The next, more highly reflective layer represents part of the photoreceptors, either the junction between the inner and outer segments (IS/OS) or the ellipsoid portion of the inner segments. The third layer likely represents the interdigitation between the RPE and photoreceptor outer segments. The outermost reflective layer represents the RPE or the RPE/Bruch's complex (Figure 4-2-2).[8] Retinal blood vessels are evident in OCT images by their shadowing of deeper retinal structures because blood is highly reflective, scattering the OCT signal. In some cases, the posterior hyaloid is visible as a thin, moderately reflective line anterior to the retina.

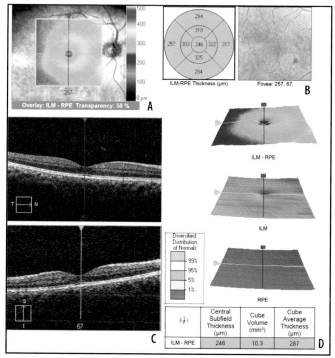

Figure 4-2-1. Macular mapping images from the Cirrus SD-OCT (Carl Zeiss Meditec). (A) A topographic map is available, as well as (B) a 9-zone Early Treatment Diabetic Retinopathy Study map and numerical thickness values. (C) Cross-sectional OCT B-scans are also displayed in both the x and y directions. The surface contour of the retina, as well as the RPE, are automatically delineated and displayed as 3-dimensional. (D) The thickness of each zone is compared with a normative database, and abnormal values are indicated with color coding: green, within normal limits; yellow, borderline; red, abnormal. Abbreviation: ILM, internal limiting membrane.

DRY AGE-RELATED MACULAR DEGENERATION: DRUSEN

On OCT, drusen are often visualized as elevations of the RPE layer and may contain materials of low, medium, or high reflectivity.[9] Drusen usually have a relatively homogeneous composition, although some drusen have a hypo- or hyperreflective core.[10] Typically, drusen elevate the RPE, and, in the case of larger soft drusen, Bruch's membrane may be visualized (Figure 4-2-3). When drusen become confluent, a retinal pigment epithelial detachment (RPED) forms, and a larger elevation of the RPE is seen. Occasionally, small subretinal spaces of hyporeflective fluid may be seen in the depressions between large, elevated drusen, which does not necessarily indicate leakage from choroidal neovascularization (CNV). Cuticular drusen (basal laminar drusen) are apparent as smaller nodular deposits below the RPE, creating a sawtooth pattern (Figure 4-2-4), whereas reticular pseudodrusen appear to be located anterior to the RPE on OCT. Often overlying drusen, the IS/OS junction and outer nuclear layer may appear thin or missing,

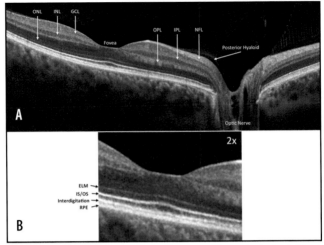

Figure 4-2-2. (A) Normal OCT. Retinal layers and the posterior hyaloid are labeled. Note the normal dip of the foveal contour. (B) A 2× magnified image of the fovea with the outer retinal layers labeled. Abbreviations: ELM, external limiting membrane; GCL, ganglion cell layer; INL, inner nuclear layer; IPL, inner plexiform layer; IS/OS, photoreceptor inner/outer segment junction; NFL, nerve fiber layer; ONL, outer nuclear layer; OPL, outer plexiform layer; RPE, retinal pigment epithelium.

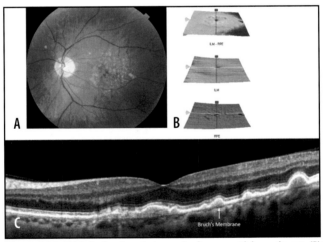

Figure 4-2-3. (A) Color fundus photograph of an eye with large drusen. (B) Reconstructed surface maps generated from OCT data show the contour of the drusen. (C) Large soft drusen elevate the RPE from Bruch's membrane and form a confluent elevation of the RPE near the fovea.

although this may not represent true damage to these layers but rather alterations in visualization of these layers due to a change in OCT light incidence on the retina.[11]

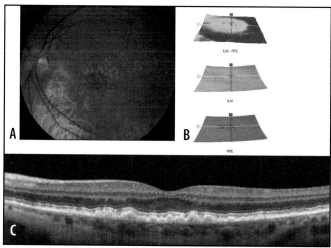

Figure 4-2-4. (A) Color fundus photograph from an eye with cuticular drusen. (B) Reconstructed surface maps from OCT data. (C) Multiple jagged or sawtooth-shaped drusen are visible. Highly reflective material is noted to elevate the RPE from Bruch's membrane.

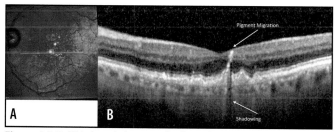

Figure 4-2-5. (A) Infrared photograph of RPE clumping. (B) On OCT, dense, highly reflective lesions are seen in the retina, representing RPE migration. Note that these lesions cause shadowing of the OCT signal past where the OCT light is incident on the lesion, demonstrating the highly backscattering nature of pigments in the RPE cells.

DRY AGE-RELATED MACULAR DEGENERATION: RETINAL PIGMENT EPITHELIUM CHANGES AND ATROPHY

In cases of focal hyperpigmentation that is apparent on examination, intraretinal migration of highly reflective RPE pigment is often visualized on OCT and may be markers of disease progression. These hyperreflective foci also may appear overlying drusen (Figure 4-2-5).[12]

Acquired vitelliform lesions can occur as a result of dry AMD and are believed to be due to RPE dysfunction. Accumulation of lipofuscin-rich material under the retina leads to the appearance of yellowish subretinal lesions. These lesions may be easily visualized on OCT as hyperreflective material in the region of the RPE, elevating the retina

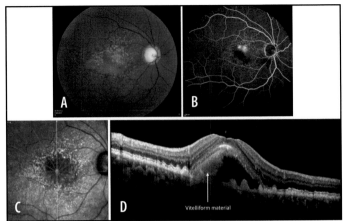

Figure 4-2-6. (A) Color fundus photograph demonstrates a vitelliform lesion and reticular pseudodrusen. This patient has reticular pseudodrusen with an associated acquired vitelliform lesion. (B) Fluorescein angiogram demonstrates an amorphous area of hyperfluorescence in the region of the vitelliform lesion, which can easily be mistaken for a CNV. (C) Infrared photograph demonstrates the orientation of the OCT scan. (D) OCT scan of the macula. The pseudodrusen are nodular and appear at the level of the RPE. The OCT scan is taken vertically and demonstrates the layering of highly reflective vitelliform material under the retina. In the superior vitelliform space, subretinal fluid is noticeable, which may be mistaken for leakage from a neovascular lesion but is likely due to resorption of the vitelliform material.

(Figure 4-2-6).[13] RPE phagocytosis of this material can lead to a fluid-filled space under the retina, which may or may not resolve over time. When this occurs, subretinal fluid is visualized on OCT, and this may sometimes be confused for active leakage of subretinal fluid from CNV.

In areas of RPE loss or detachment, Bruch's membrane becomes visible, and in areas of RPE loss, the OCT signal is able to penetrate into the choroid and sclera more readily. On OCT, areas of RPE atrophy appear as focal thinning of the RPE layer, resulting in areas of increased penetration of OCT signal into the underlying choriocapillaris and sclera (Figure 4-2-7).[14] The demarcation of healthy and atrophic RPE is often abrupt. Overlying areas of RPE atrophy, the inner retinal layers, including the IS/OS junction, as well as the outer nuclear layer, may appear thinned or missing. On occasion, retinal pseudocysts may appear overlying areas of geographic atrophy (GA), which likely represent a degenerative process within the retina.[15] However, in the transition zone between healthy and diseased RPE, the photoreceptor layers (IS/OS, ELM) may sometimes taper off, and the RPE height may appear increased or decreased, suggesting abnormalities in the structure of the retina in this transition zone.[16]

In addition, a form of dry age-related maculopathy has been described using EDI-OCT: age-related choroidal atrophy. These patients present with symptoms out of proportion to clinical findings, which are typically mild to moderate diffuse changes of dry AMD. On EDI-OCT, many of these patients have a dramatically thin choroid compared with the normal thinning of the choroid that occurs with age.[17] It remains to be seen whether this might be a distinct disease entity or a subgroup of AMD.

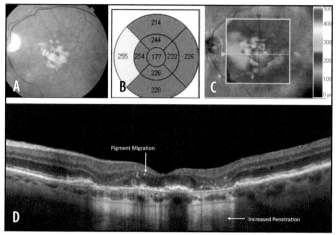

Figure 4-2-7. (A) Color fundus photograph demonstrates GA. (B) The retina is thinner than normal and appears red on the Early Treatment Diabetic Retinopathy Study map when compared with a normative database. (C) Thickness map generated from OCT data demonstrates thinning of the macula. (D) OCT image of the macula. Where the RPE is missing, OCT signal can penetrate more easily into the choroid and sclera. As well as the RPE, the photoreceptor layers also degenerate and disappear over areas of GA. This patient may have good vision because of a central island of preserved photoreceptors and RPE.

WET AGE-RELATED MACULAR DEGENERATION

Neovascular, or wet, AMD is caused by the growth of abnormal vessels in the macula. These vessels are highly permeable, and resultant leakage can lead to the accumulation of fluid, hemorrhage, and exudates under the RPE, under the retina, and within the retina. Because OCT is extremely sensitive at detecting the microscopic details of these abnormalities, it can help to determine the exact location of fluid accumulation and can quantify changes in fluid over time. On OCT, fluid appears hyporeflective. If fluid occurs under the RPE, a serous RPED forms. When fluid accumulates under the retina, a serous neurosensory detachment can be visualized. Fluid in the retina may also accumulate, which appears as small, round hyporeflective cystic spaces within the retina on OCT. Hard exudates are also visible on OCT and appear as small highly reflective lesions, typically within the outer retina. Hemorrhage is also highly reflective and appears as amorphous material under the RPE, under the retina, or within the retina.

In addition, OCT is able to visualize CNV, the primary lesion in wet AMD. CNVs that appear classic (type 2) on fluorescein angiography are visualized as hyperreflective lesions anterior to the RPE, whereas occult (type 1) CNVs appear as hyperreflective lesions underneath the RPE (Figure 4-2-8).[18] Type 1 CNVs may create a fibrovascular RPED, an elevation of the RPE by material of variable optical density on OCT (depending on the fibrous, fluid, and/or neovascular composition). Analysis by EDI-OCT of the internal characteristics of fibrovascular RPEDs secondary to AMD has demonstrated that the CNV proliferates along the undersurface of the RPED.[19] Types 1 and 2 CNV may be difficult to distinguish from hemorrhage on OCT because both hemorrhage and CNVs are highly reflective, and clinical correlation is often helpful to differentiate the

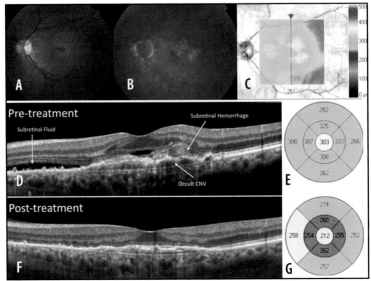

Figure 4-2-8. (A) Color fundus photograph shows pigment changes and drusen. (B) Fluorescein angiogram shows late ill-defined leakage consistant with an occult CNV. (C) Macular thickness map constructed from OCT data shows slight thickening (yellow) of the macula. (D) OCT shows an occult CNV, which appears underneath the RPE, as a broad-based, ill-defined neovascular network that elevates the RPE from Bruch's membrane. A small subretinal hemorrhage is present, which is highly reflective and ill-defined. Subretinal fluid is present. (E) Early Treatment Diabetic Retinopathy Study map shows mild thickening of the center circle. (F) OCT shows that after treatment with anti-VEGF medication, the fluid and hemorrhage resolve. (G) After treatment, the thickness on the Early Treatment Diabetic Retinopathy Study map decreases.

two. Contraction of the CNV has been associated with the formation of RPE tears, which may occur as part of the natural history of the disease. These tears are visible on OCT as an abrupt disruption of the RPE line; the RPE often appears elevated and scrolled where the tear occured.[20]

Retinal angiomatous proliferation (RAP), or type 3 CNV, occurs when there is an anastamosis between abnormal vessels within the retina and under the RPE. On OCT, RAP lesions are characterized by a fibrovascular RPED in association with significant accumulations of intraretinal fluid (although these 2 findings in conjunction are not pathognomonic of RAP) (Figure 4-2-9).[21] Occasionally, the abnormal retinal vessels of the RAP lesion may be visualized using OCT.

Polypoidal choroidal vasculopathy (PCV) likely comes in 2 varieties: a distinct disease (found in a younger age group than is typical of AMD and without other fundus findings typical of AMD) and as a subset of wet AMD. In PCV, patients develop multiple serosanguinous RPEDs caused by sub-RPE branching neovascular networks containing characteristic polypoidal lesions, which are best seen with indocyanine green angiography. On OCT, the branching neovascular networks can be seen between Bruch's membrane and the RPE, elevating the RPE in broad irregular patches, whereas polypoidal lesions cause more discrete RPE elevations.[22] Serous or hemorrhagic RPEDs can often be seen adjacent to the neovascular PCV lesions (Figure 4-2-10). Subfoveal choroidal thickness

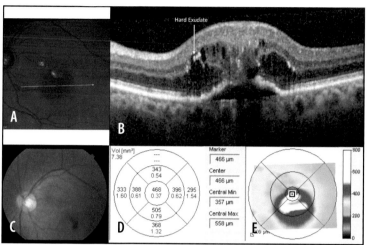

Figure 4-2-9. (A) Infrared image shows the orientation of the OCT image through a macular RAP lesion. (B) An RAP lesion occurs when abnormal retinal and choroidal vessels form an anastamosis. This is apparent on OCT as a large pigment epithelial detachment, as well as intraretinal fluid, hemorrhage, and exudate. Exudates are highly reflective, small intraretinal lesions. (C) Color fundus photograph shows a small intraretinal hemorrhage. (D) Early Treatment Diabetic Retinopathy Study map from the OCT data shows thickening of the center circle. (E) Macular thickness map from OCT data shows thickening of the central macula (red and white).

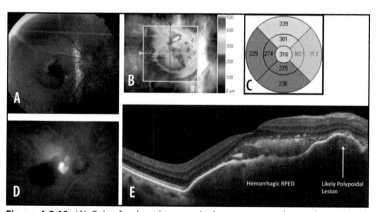

Figure 4-2-10. (A) Color fundus photograph demonstrates submacular and sub-RPE hemorrhage, consistent with PCV. (B) Macular thickness map from OCT data demonstrates macular thickening due to subretinal fluid and hemorrhage. (C) Early Treatment Diabetic Retinopathy map from OCT data demonstrates thickening of the macula. (D) Indocyanine green angiography image demonstrates focal hyperfluorescent polypoid lesions and adjacent RPED. (E) OCT demonstrates a hemorrhagic RPED, as well as subretinal hemorrhage. Polypoidal lesions are evident on OCT as more focal elevations of the RPE.

on EDI-OCT has been shown to be increased in patients with PCV in comparison with other forms of wet AMD.[23]

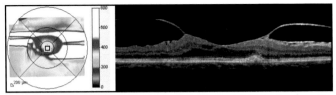

Figure 4-2-11. Segmentation artifact. When the hyaloid detaches from the retina, it can cause automated segmentation software to malfunction. This causes abrupt changes in macular thickness measurements, seen on the macular thickness map as artificial square or spoke-like patterns.

The end-stage lesion of wet AMD is a disciform scar. This occurs when subretinal fibrosis overtakes the neovascular component of a CNV membrane, damaging the retina and RPE and resulting in poor visual acuity. These fibrotic scars appear highly reflective on OCT and are typically well-circumscribed.[2]

AGE-RELATED MACULAR DEGENERATION AND THE VITREOMACULAR INTERFACE

As the vitreous becomes more liquefied with age, it starts to separate from the macula. This separation of the posterior hyaloid membrane from the macula can be visualized on OCT, and vitreomacular attachment is often not pathologic. However, when the vitreomacular adhesion is abnormally strong (or if liquefication of the vitreous outpaces vitreomacular separation), vitreomacular traction (VMT) ensues, leading to distortion and thickening of the macula, resulting in blurred and distorted vision (Figure 4-2-11). Studies suggest that patients with wet AMD have a higher incidence of vitreomacular traction than those without wet AMD and that VMT may have some role in macular thickening and visual distortion in select patients with wet AMD.[24] However, further prospective studies are needed to corroborate these findings.

MACULAR MAPS AND PATIENT MONITORING

Since the introduction of commercially available OCT devices, one of the key features of OCT has been the ability to calculate macular thickness using automated software algorithms. Older TD-OCT devices used only a few scans through the macula to calculate these maps, but newer SD-OCT devices can calculate detailed macular thickness maps with greater precision using a much greater wealth of data. Macular maps are a useful way to monitor patients with AMD because they can provide precise numerical values of macular thicknesses that can be followed over time or after treatment. Notably, macular maps are calculated by automated software that can break down; therefore, care must be taken to ensure that no software-related artifacts are present (discussed later in this section).

With the advent of anti-VEGF intravitreal injection treatments for AMD, OCT has become the gold standard for following treatment response (see Figure 4-2-8). Both macular maps and individual images can be used to assess the presence or absence of fluid on OCT, which is the main indicator of neovascular activity. In several prospective studies, including the Comparison of Age-Related Macular Degeneration Treatment Trial

(CATT)[25] and the HARBOR trial,[26] OCT was used as the main indicator of whether to treat or not treat patients (patients with any sign of intra- or subretinal fluid on OCT were treated), and most retinal specialists use OCT as the primary tool in directing decision making when it comes to anti-VEGF therapy.

LIMITATIONS AND ARTIFACTS

As with any imaging modality, OCT has some limitations. OCT measures changes in optical properties within tissue, which do not necessarily directly correlate to anatomic structures seen on histology examination. OCT can be limited by media opacities such as cataracts or vitreous hemorrhage. OCT also depends on operator skill. The operator must take each image in range and in focus, and the scan must be examined for blinks and motion artifacts. Poor-quality scans should be discarded and repeated by the operator. Patient motion in the axial direction can be corrected with computer software; however, transverse motion cannot be corrected. The operator is also responsible for centering the images at the fovea. This can be difficult in patients with AMD because the foveal contour can be distorted. Patients with AMD may also have trouble with fixation, and external fixation with the contralateral eye may be used in these patients.

The use of computer algorithms to determine retinal thickness also introduces artifacts. In patients with AMD, the outer retinal boundary may become unclear if altered by drusen, RPEDs, or CNV. If the posterior hyaloid is visible, automated software may mistakenly measure the hyaloid as the inner retinal boundary. Segmentation artifacts can be observed in individual OCT images, or they can be visualized on the macular map as abrupt nonphysiologic changes in macular thickness (see Figure 4-2-10). Errors of segmentation also can occur in scans with lower signal-to-noise ratios, and most clinically available OCT devices offer a signal strength measurement to determine the quality of each OCT scan.

SUMMARY

OCT is an imaging device capable of unparalleled high-resolution imaging of the macula. Individual OCT scans allow for analysis of macular anatomy in microscopic detail, whereas the thickness mapping capabilities of OCT make it a useful tool in managing patients over time. In both nonexudative and exudative AMD, OCT allows for precise visualization of macular pathologies, including drusen, GA, abnormalities of the RPE, and CNV. In wet AMD, OCT has become the gold standard to monitor patients who receive intravitreal injections of anti-VEGF medication. OCT has now become an essential tool in the diagnosis and management of patients with AMD and a virtual necessity in today's retinal practice.

REFERENCES

1. Huang D, Swanson EA, Lin CP, et al. Optical coherence tomography. *Science*. 1991;254(5035):1178-1181.
2. Keane PA, Patel PJ, Liakopoulos S, Heussen FM, Sadda SR, Tufail A. Evaluation of age-related macular degeneration with optical coherence tomography. *Surv Ophthalmol*. 2012;57(5):389-414.
3. Hee MR, Izatt JA, Swanson EA, et al. Optical coherence tomography of the human retina. *Arch Ophthalmol*. 1995;113(3):325-332.

4. Drexler W, Morgner U, Ghanta RK, Kartner FX, Schuman JS, Fujimoto JG. Ultrahigh-resolution ophthalmic optical coherence tomography. *Nat Med.* 2001;7(4):502-507.

5. Wojtkowski M, Bajraszewski T, Gorczynska I, et al. Ophthalmic imaging by spectral optical coherence tomography. *Am J Ophthalmol.* 2004;138(3):412-419.

6. Spaide RF, Koizumi H, Pozzoni MC. Enhanced depth imaging spectral-domain optical coherence tomography. *Am J Ophthalmol.* 2008;146(4):496-500.

7. Anger EM, Unterhuber A, Hermann B, et al. Ultrahigh resolution optical coherence tomography of the monkey fovea. Identification of retinal sublayers by correlation with semithin histology sections. *Exp Eye Res.* 2004;78(6):1117-1125.

8. Srinivasan VJ, Monson BK, Wojtkowski M, et al. Characterization of outer retinal morphology with high-speed, ultrahigh-resolution optical coherence tomography. *Invest Ophthalmol Vis Sci.* 2008;49(4):1571-1579.

9. Spaide RF, Curcio CA. Drusen characterization with multimodal imaging. *Retina.* 2010;30:1441-1454.

10. Leuschen JN, Schuman SG, Winter KP, et al. Spectral-domain optical coherence tomography characteristics of intermediate age-related macular degeneration. *Ophthalmology.* 2013;120(1):140-150.

11. Schuman S, Koreishi A, Farsiu S, et al. Photoreceptor layer thinning over drusen in eyes with age-related macular degeneration imaged in vivo with spectral- domain optical coherence tomography. *Ophthalmology.* 2009;116:488-496.

12. Christenbury JG, Folgar FA, O'Connell RV, et al. Progression of intermediate age-related macular degeneration with proliferation and Inner retinal migration of hyperreflective foci. *Ophthalmology.* 2013;120(5):1038-1045.

13. Freund KB, Laud K, Lima LH, et al. Acquired vitelliform lesions: correlation of clinical findings and multiple imaging analyses. *Retina.* 2011;31:13-25.

14. Wolf-Schnurrbusch UEK, Enzmann V, Brinkmann CK, et al. Morphologic changes in patients with geographic atrophy assessed with a novel spectral OCT-SLO combination. *Invest Ophthalmol Vis Sci.* 2008;49:3095-3099.

15. Cohen SY, Dubois L, Nghiem-Buffet S, et al. Retinal pseudocysts in age-related geographic atrophy. *Am J Ophthalmol.* 2010;150(2):211-217.

16. Bearelly S, Chau FY, Koreishi A, Stinnett SS, Izatt JA, Toth CA. Spectral domain optical coherence tomography imaging of geographic atrophy margins. *Ophthalmology.* 2009;116(9):1762-1769.

17. Spaide RF. Age-related choroidal atrophy. *Am J Ophthalmol.* 2009;147:801-810.

18. Hughes EH, Khan J, Patel N, et al. In vivo demonstration of the anatomic differences between classic and occult choroidal neovascularization using optical coherence tomography. *Am J Ophthalmol.* 2005;139:344-346.

19. Spaide RF. Enhanced depth imaging optical coherence tomography of retinal pigment epithelial detachment in age-related macular degeneration. *Am J Ophthalmol.* 2009;147(4):644-652.

20. Chan CK, Meyer CH, Gross JG, et al. Retinal pigment epithelial tears after intravitreal bevacizumab injection for neovascular age-related macular degeneration. *Retina.* 2007;27(5):541-551.

21. Truong SN, Alam S, Zawadzki RJ, et al. High resolution Fourier-domain optical coherence tomography of retinal angiomatous proliferation. *Retina.* 2007;27:915-925.

22. Ojima Y, Hangai M, Sakamoto A, et al. Improved visualization of polypoidal choroidal vasculopathy lesions using spectral-domain optical coherence tomography. *Retina.* 2009;29(1):52-59.

23. Chung SE, Kang SW, Lee JH, Kim YT. Choroidal thickness in polypoidal choroidal vasculopathy and exudative age-related macular degeneration. *Ophthalmology.* 2011;118(5):840-845.

24. Krebs I, Brannath W, Glittenberg C, et al. Posterior vitreomacular adhesion: a potential risk factor for exudative age-related macular degeneration? *Am J Ophthalmol.* 2007;144:741-746.

25. Comparison of Age-related Macular Degeneration Treatments Trials (CATT) Research Group, Martin DF, Maguire MG, et al. Ranibizumab and bevacizumab for treatment of neovascular age-related macular degeneration: two-year results. *Ophthalmology.* 2012;119(7):1388-1398.

26. Busbee BG, Ho AC, Brown DM, et al. Twelve-month efficacy and safety of 0.5 mg or 2.0 mg ranibizumab in patients with subfoveal neovascular age-related macular degeneration. *Ophthalmology.* 2013;120(5):1046-1056.

4

SECTION 3: FLUORESCEIN ANGIOGRAPHY AND INDOCYANINE GREEN ANGIOGRAPHY

Michael D. Tibbetts, MD and Elias Reichel, MD

Fluorescein angiography (FA) and indocyanine green angiography (ICGA) are important testing modalities to diagnose age-related macular degeneration (AMD).[1] These technologies use intravenous dyes that facilitate imaging of the circulation of the retina and choroid. FA was developed and quickly became widely used in the 1970s for the study of AMD after the work of Gass.[2] ICGA was also developed in the 1970s, but its clinical use did not begin until the 1990s with the introduction of digital imaging systems to acquire clinically meaningful images.[3-7] FA is still considered the gold standard for diagnosing choroidal neovascularization (CNV), even in the era of high-resolution optical coherence tomography (OCT; see Chapter 4, Section 2).[8] ICGA excels at imaging the deep structure of the choroidal vasculature and is useful to differentiate AMD from other related diseases of the retinal pigment epithelium and choroid.[9]

FLUORESCEIN ANGIOGRAPHY

Technique

To perform FA, sodium fluorescein in a sterile aqueous solution (25% concentration in 2 to 3 mL, or 10%, concentration in 5 mL) is injected intravenously. The majority of fluorescein is protein-bound, and the remaining 20% circulates in the vasculature, including the tissues of the retina and choroid. Sodium fluorescein fluoresces at a wavelength of 520 to 535 nm (green) after excitation by light of 485 to 500 nm (blue). White light from a camera flash is passed through a blue filter, which then excites the unbound fluorescein molecules circulating in the retinal and choroidal blood vessels or those that have leaked out of the vasculature. The blue light stimulates the fluorescein molecule to emit longer-wavelength, yellow-green light. The emitted fluorescence and reflected blue light return to the camera, where a yellow-green filter blocks the reflected blue light and allows only the yellow-green fluorescence to enter the camera, where it is captured onto film or a digital surface. The standard angle of view is 30 degrees with 2.5× magnification. Wide-field FA permits viewing angles of up to 200 degrees to image the peripheral retina.

The side effects of FA in all patients include yellowing of the skin and conjunctiva for 2 to 6 hours and fluorescent urine for 1 to 2 days. More concerning side effects can include nausea, vomiting, or vasovagal reactions in 5% to 10% of patients, urticarial reactions in 1%, and rare anaphylactic reactions (fewer than 1 in 100,000).[10]

Interpretation

FAs are interpreted based on the pattern, timing, and location of the fluorescence. Hypofluorescence occurs when the fluorescence signal is blocked by overlying pigment, blood, or fibrous tissue or if the blood vessels do not fill properly, resulting in a vascular filling defect. Hyperfluorescence can be seen in several major patterns, including leakage, staining, pooling, and transmission or window defects, all of which may occur in patients with AMD. Leakage describes the gradual, marked increase in fluorescence throughout the FA as the fluorescein molecules diffuse through the retinal pigment epithelium (RPE) into the subretinal space, out of blood vessels, or from retinal neovascularization into the vitreous. In contrast, staining denotes a pattern of fluorescence when fluorescein enters a solid tissue, such as a scar or drusen. The fluorescence pattern of staining demonstrates a gradual increase in intensity into the late views, with fixed borders that do not expand. Pooling describes the accumulation of fluorescein in a fluid-filled space in the retina or choroid, as in a detachment of the RPE. Finally, a transmission, or window defect, refers to a view of the normal choroidal fluorescence through a defect in the pigment or loss of the RPE.

Fluorescein Angiography of Dry Age-Related Macular Degeneration

The FA findings in non-neovascular (dry) AMD are characterized by alterations in the RPE and Bruch's membrane that are the hallmark of the disease. The most typical findings of dry AMD are drusen, which may stain in late views (Figure 4-3-1). Fluorescein may also pool in areas of diffuse thickening of Bruch's membrane that are characterized by soft, confluent drusen. FA may demonstrate more numerous drusen in patients with basal laminar drusen with a "starry sky" appearance and may show leakage into the subretinal space within a pseudovitelliform detachment (Figure 4-3-2). Retinal pigment epithelial detachments (RPEDs) may fill rapidly with fluorescein as the dye leaks out of the choriocapillaris and pools within the area of the RPEDs. Areas of geographic atrophy (GA) in which the RPE is either absent or attenuated will demonstrate a characteristic window defect on FA (Figures 4-3-3 and 4-3-4). Focal areas of hyperpigmentation due to alterations in the RPE may cause a blockage defect.

Fluorescein Angiography of Wet Age-Related Macular Degeneration

FA is the gold standard for diagnosing CNV, the hallmark lesion of neovascular (wet) AMD.[8] If wet AMD is suspected based on the fundus appearance or other findings, FA should be obtained and interpreted. OCT plays an important role in AMD diagnosis and treatment decisions (see Chapter 4, Section 2), but in a prospective study, time-domain OCT was only moderately sensitive (0.69 compared with FA as the gold standard) with high specificity.[11] Higher-resolution spectral-domain OCT likely has higher sensitivity

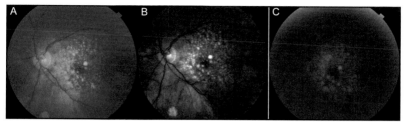

Figure 4-3-1. Staining of drusen on FA. (A) Color fundus photograph shows numerous medium and large drusen in the macula in a patient with dry AMD. (B) Red-free photograph demonstrates bright drusen. (C) Late-phase FA shows staining of drusen, with no evidence of CNV.

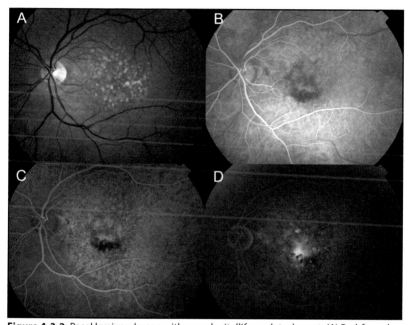

Figure 4-3-2. Basal laminar drusen with pseudovitelliform detachment. (A) Red-free photograph shows numerous well-defined drusen and shallow subretinal fluid in the central macula. (B) Laminar venous-phase FA shows early leakage into the subretinal space of the pseudovitelliform detachment in the central macula and highlights the basal laminar drusen. (C) Arteriovenous-phase FA highlights the basal laminar drusen with a "starry sky" appearance and shows increased leakage of subretinal fluid. (D) Late-phase FA shows staining of drusen and increased leakage into the pseudovitelliform detachment.

in detecting new-onset CNV; however, there continues to be a role for FA in the diagnosis of AMD and the detection of new-onset CNV.

FA patterns of CNV vary based on the size of the CNV and the anatomic and vascular alterations to Bruch's membrane, the RPE, and neurosensory retina. Landmark clinical trials, including the Macular Photocoagulation Study (MPS), defined the location of CNV as *extrafoveal, subfoveal,* or *juxtafoveal*.[12,13] *Extrafoveal* CNV can be found between 200 and 2500 µm from the geometric center of the foveal avascular zone (FAZ). *Juxtafoveal* CNV are located up to 199 µm from the FAZ center and may include portions of the FAZ

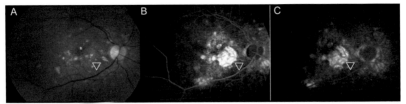

Figure 4-3-3. Multifocal GA in a patient with dry AMD. (A) Color fundus photograph shows numerous drusen and multiple areas of GA with largest area marked by an arrowhead. (B) Recirculation-phase FA demonstrates well-defined area of hyperfluorescence (arrowhead) from choroidal circulation corresponding to an area of GA. (C) Late-phase FA shows persistent hyperfluorescence in an area of GA, with relative hypofluorescence of choroidal vessels and no evidence of leakage.

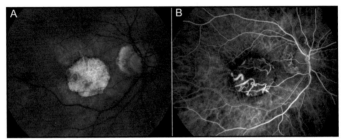

Figure 4-3-4. GA in a patient with age-related choroidal atrophy. (A) Color fundus photograph shows a large area of GA in the central macula and peripapillary atrophy. (B) Laminar venous-phase FA demonstrates a large area of GA in the central macula, with a window defect allowing visualization of the underlying choroidal vasculature.

but not the center. *Subfoveal* CNV are contiguous with the area directly beneath the center of the FAZ. These definitions were particularly important to determine the prognosis and feasibility of treatment with laser photocoagulation of CNV in the era before anti-vascular endothelial growth factor (anti-VEGF) therapy (see Chapter 7).

The 2 major patterns of CNV on FA have historically been described as *classic* and *occult*.[13] A classic, or type 2, CNV is characterized by a fairly well-defined area of hyperfluorescence seen in the early phase of the FA that progressively intensifies throughout the transit phase, with leakage of fluorescein obscuring the boundaries of the lesion by the late phases (Figure 4-3-5). Anatomically, type 2 CNV membranes are located above the RPE. An occult, or type 1, CNV is seen in early frames as mottled and patchy early hyperfluorescence with poorly defined borders that leak in later frames to form a larger area of stippled, irregular hyperfluorescence (Figure 4-3-6). Type 1 CNV membranes are located below the RPE. Occult CNV has been described in 2 forms: as a fibrovascular RPED or as late leakage from an undetermined source. A fibrovascular RPED describes an area of stippled or granular fluorescence that typically fills within 1 to 2 minutes after fluorescein injection. In contrast, late leakage from an undetermined source denotes late fluorescence at the level of the RPE, which does not correspond to an RPE elevation or a classic CNV. A third type of neovascularization in AMD, known as *retinal angiomatous proliferation* (RAP), or type 3 CNV, is associated with proliferation of new vessels within the retina itself.[14] RAP lesions typically exhibit indistinct staining on FA similar

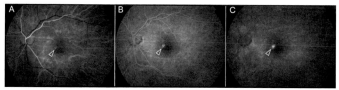

Figure 4-3-5. Classic CNV. (A) Arterial-phase FA shows early hypofluorescence nasal to the fovea (arrowhead). (B) Arteriovenous-phase FA demonstrates increased hyperfluorescence in a well-defined pattern, consistent with classic CNV. (C) Late-phase FA shows late leakage of classic CNV.

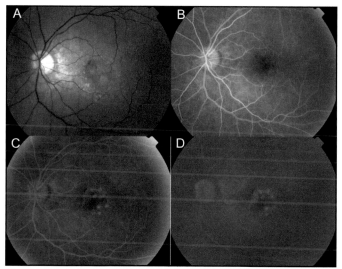

Figure 4-3-6. Occult CNV. (A) Red-free photograph shows drusen, hemorrhage, and shallow elevation of the RPE in the central macula. (B) Arteriovenous-phase FA reveals faint patchy hyperfluorescence in the central macula. (C) Recirculation-phase FA shows increasing patchy and poorly defined areas of hyperfluorescence. (D) Late-phase FA shows increasing patchy hyperfluorescence with leakage.

to occult CNV and are differentiated based on the finding of intense focal hyperfluorescence on ICGA.

The differentiation of these patterns was particularly important with regard to the efficacy of laser photocoagulation and verteporfin photodynamic therapy (PDT). In the clinical trials of PDT, namely the Treatment of AMD With Photodynamic Therapy (TAP) study and Verteporfin in Photodynamic Therapy (VIP) study, a further differentiation was made between *predominantly classic*, *minimally classic*, and *occult with no classic* CNV based on FA.[15,16] These studies included patients with subfoveal CNV no greater than 5400 µm in linear diameter. Predominantly classic CNV occupy more than 50% of the entire lesion with the classic pattern. Minimally classic CNV is defined by a classic CNV that occupies 1% to 49% of the entire lesion. Occult with no classic CNV contains only occult CNV. In the TAP study, patients with predominantly classic lesions showed a benefit from PDT compared with placebo.[15] In contrast, the VIP study demonstrated no benefit for occult CNV at one year into the study but showed a small benefit to PDT at 2 years after treatment.[16] The initial hypothesis that the prognosis of CNV lesions that consist solely of occult CNV may be better than lesions consisting of classic CNV or a mixture of classic and occult CNV was not proven by a meta-analysis of untreated eyes from clinical trials.[17] Instead, the final visual acuity was independent of the FA classification and was primarily determined by the initial visual acuity. In addition to its role in diagnosis, FA can also be used to monitor treatment response. The disappearance of leakage on FA can indicate regression of CNV, whereas new leakage can indicate recurrence.[1]

FA is also useful to diagnose and characterize RPEDs, which occur commonly in AMD, as well as other diseases of the choroid, including central serous chorioretinopathy (CSC). RPEDs can be described as *serous, fibrovascular,* or *drusenoid*.[18] A serous RPED is characterized by rapid, early, homogenous, and intense fluorescence that retains its boundaries and intensity throughout the FA. The intense fluorescence is due to the diffusion of fluorescein across a permeable Bruch's membrane, with pooling in the sub-RPE space. In contrast to a serous RPED, a fibrovascular RPED, which is a subset of occult CNV (as mentioned previously), has irregular topography of the RPE elevation, a stippled and nonhomogenous pattern of fluorescence, and a slow rate of filling. Serous RPEDs fluoresce between 20 and 60 seconds after fluorescein injection, whereas fibrovascular RPEDs fluoresce between 1 and 3 minutes, with either leakage or staining in the late phase. Drusenoid RPEDs are formed by the progressive enlargement and confluence of soft drusen.[19] On FA, there is gradual staining of the sub-RPE space, with no leakage or irregular density as the fluorescein enters the confluent drusen, but it does not pool or leak.

Differentiation of Age-Related Macular Degeneration From Other Diseases Based on Fluorescein Angiography Findings

FA may be useful to differentiate AMD from a number of disease mimickers or masquerade conditions, including pattern dystrophy, CSC, idiopathic uveal effusion syndrome, and PCV (see Chapter 5). Pattern dystrophy is a condition defined by focal pinpoint or reticular hyperpigmentation surrounded by a vitelliform detachment with a characteristic yellowish abnormality of the outer retina. On FA, late staining of the vitelliform detachment may help distinguish pattern dystrophy from AMD. FA is also helpful to differentiate AMD from other entities that may cause subretinal fluid, including CSC, optic nerve pits, PCV, and idiopathic uveal effusion syndrome. The area of subretinal fluid associated with CNV and PCV usually corresponds closely to the area of leakage on FA, in contrast to the characteristic pinpoint leak relative to a large area of subretinal fluid in CSC. The pattern of leakage in idiopathic uveal effusion syndrome is usually diffuse, with more prominent subretinal fluid.

INDOCYANINE GREEN ANGIOGRAPHY

Technique

Indocyanine green (ICG) is a water-soluble, high-molecular-weight dye that fluoresces with a peak absorption of 805 nm and peak emission of 835 nm.[9] The dye is almost completely protein bound, which limits its diffusion through the small fenestrations of

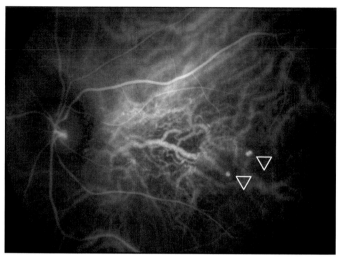

Figure 4-3-7. ICGA demonstrates 2 discrete areas of hyperfluorescence (arrowheads), consistent with vascular polyps characteristic of PCV.

the choriocapillaris; thereby, the dye remains in the choroidal circulation. A confocal laser illumination system induces fluorescence from the ICG molecule, and specialized infrared video angiography, typically using a scanning laser ophthalmoscope, detects the fluorescence. Given the different wavelengths of fluorescence, modern imaging systems can obtain FA and ICGA images simultaneously. The theoretical advantage of ICGA, given the longer infrared wavelength, compared with fluorescein is the ability to fluoresce through opacities, including pigment, fluid, lipid, and blood. These properties allow for improved imaging of occult CNV and RPEDs.[4,20] In addition, the scanning laser ophthalmoscope imaging system focuses infrared light on a narrow area of the retinal surface, thereby allowing greater contrast than conventional fundus images.[21]

ICG has a lower rate of side effects compared with fluorescein, although allergic reactions can be more severe. Mild adverse events, including nausea, vomiting, sneezing, and itching, occur in 0.15% of cases.[22] More severe reactions, including urticaria, syncope, hypotension, and anaphylaxis, are rare. Allergic reactions are extremely rare, but ICG should be used with caution in individuals with an iodide or shellfish allergy because the dye contains 5% iodide. Given that ICG is metabolized in the liver, the test should be avoided in individuals with hepatic disease.

Interpretation and Indications

The interpretation of ICGA is based on the pattern, location, and timing of the imaged fluorescence. CNV manifests on ICGA as a plaque, focal hot spot, or a combination of both.[23,24] Plaques are usually formed by late-staining vessels and may correspond to occult CNV. In contrast, focal hot spots are well-defined areas of hyperfluorescence less than one disc diameter in size that may indicate RAPs or polypoidal CNV (Figure 4-3-7).[23] ICGA provides the necessary contrast to distinguish RAP lesions from occult or minimally classic CNV because the dye does not leak into the subretinal or sub-RPE space.[14]

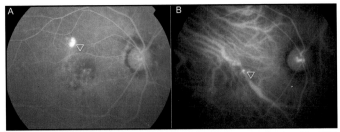

Figure 4-3-8. Comparison of FA and ICGA in a patient with PCV. (A) Recirculation-phase FA demonstrates a well-defined area of hyperfluorescence (arrowhead) in the superior macula, consistent with CNV. (B) ICGA shows a punctate area of hyperfluorescence, consistent with a vascular polyp that is characteristic of PCV.

One of the most important uses of ICG is to differentiate wet AMD from PCV (Figure 4-3-8).[25] Yannuzzi[5] proposed that ICGA should be used for suspected wet AMD with any of 5 features that are more common in PCV:

- Darkly pigmented patients
- Serosanguineous macular detachment in the peripapillary area
- Serosanguineous macular detachment in the absence of drusen
- Large, vascularized RPED, particularly with extensive blood or lipid or minimal cystoid macular edema
- Vascularized RPED, which has proven resistant or minimally responsive to multiple anti-VEGF injections

ICG can also be useful to distinguish atypical diffuse CSC in older patients from occult choroidal CNV in AMD. ICGA may demonstrate the characteristic multifocal hyperfluorescent patches associated with choroidal hyperpermeability in CSC. ICGA may also be particularly helpful to identify recurrent CNV after laser photocoagulation where the margins of the original lesion have been obscured.[26] Early studies also used ICGA to identify the feeder vessels of CNV for treatment with laser photocoagulation.[27,28] The results of these early studies were mixed, and the technique did not gain wide acceptance because the availability of photodynamic therapy and anti-VEGF agents soon replaced laser photocoagulation for many indications.

SUMMARY

FA is useful in characterizing AMD and is still the gold standard used to diagnose wet AMD. FA can be used to categorize types of CNV in AMD and to guide laser treatment (thermal laser or PDT) of CNV membranes. ICGA can be used to detect certain subtypes of wet AMD, such as PCV and RAP, or to differentiate AMD from some mimickers of the disease, such as CSC. Both FA and ICGA remain important diagnostic tools in the clinical management of AMD.

REFERENCES

1.   Gess AJ, Fung AE, Rodriguez JG. Imaging in neovascular age-related macular degeneration. *Semin Ophthalmol.* 2011;26:225-233.

2. Gass JD. Drusen and disciform macular detachment and degeneration. *Trans Am Ophthalmol Soc.* 1972;70:409-436.

3. Guyer DR, Puliafito CA, Mones JM, Friedman E, Chang W, Verdooner SR. Digital indocyanine-green angiography in chorioretinal disorders. *Ophthalmology.* 1992;99:287-291.

4. Yannuzzi LA, Slakter JS, Sorenson JA, Guyer DR, Orlock DA. Digital indocyanine green videoangiography and choroidal neovascularization. *Retina.* 1992;12:191-223.

5. Yannuzzi LA. Indocyanine green angiography: a perspective on use in the clinical setting. *Am J Ophthalmol.* 2011;151:745-751.e1.

6. Flower RW, Hochheimer BF. Indocyanine green dye fluorescence and infrared absorption choroidal angiography performed simultaneously with fluorescein angiography. *Johns Hopkins Med J.* 1976;138:33-42.

7. Orth DH, Patz A, Flower RW. Potential clinical applications of indocyanine green choroidal angiography: preliminary report. *Eye Ear Nose Throat Mon.* 1976;55:15-28, 58.

8. Do DV. Detection of new-onset choroidal neovascularization. *Curr Opin Ophthalmol.* 2013;24:244-247.

9. Reichel E, Puliafito CA. *Atlas of Indocyanine Green Angiography.* New York, NY: Igaku-Shoin Medical Publishers Inc; 1996.

10. Kwiterovich KA, Maguire MG, Murphy RP, et al. Frequency of adverse systemic reactions after fluorescein angiography. Results of a prospective study. *Ophthalmology.* 1991;98:1139-1142.

11. Do DV, Gower EW, Cassard SD, et al. Detection of new-onset choroidal neovascularization using optical coherence tomography: the AMD DOC Study. *Ophthalmology.* 2012;119:771-778.

12. Argon laser photocoagulation for senile macular degeneration. Results of a randomized clinical trial. *Arch Ophthalmol.* 1982;100:912-918.

13. Argon laser photocoagulation for neovascular maculopathy. Three-year results from randomized clinical trials. Macular Photocoagulation Study Group. *Arch Ophthalmol.* 1986;104:694-701.

14. Yannuzzi LA, Negrao S, Iida T, et al. Retinal angiomatous proliferation in age-related macular degeneration. *Retina.* 2001;21:416-434.

15. Photodynamic therapy of subfoveal choroidal neovascularization in age-related macular degeneration with verteporfin: one-year results of 2 randomized clinical trials—TAP report. Treatment of age-related macular degeneration with photodynamic therapy (TAP) Study Group. *Arch Ophthalmol.* 1999;117:1329-1345.

16. Verteporfin in Photodynamic Therapy Study Group. Verteporfin therapy of subfoveal choroidal neovascularization in age-related macular degeneration: two-year results of a randomized clinical trial including lesions with occult with no classic choroidal neovascularization—verteporfin in photodynamic therapy report 2. *Am J Ophthalmol.* 2001;131(5):541-560.

17. Shah AR, Del Priore LV. Natural history of predominantly classic, minimally classic, and occult subgroups in exudative age-related macular degeneration. *Ophthalmology.* 2009;116:1901-1907.

18. Zayit-Soudry S, Moroz I, Loewenstein A. Retinal pigment epithelial detachment. *Surv Ophthalmol.* 2007;52:227-243.

19. Roquet W, Roudot-Thoraval F, Coscas G, Soubrane G. Clinical features of drusenoid pigment epithelial detachment in age-related macular degeneration. *Br J Ophthalmol.* 2004;88:638-642.

20. Reichel E, Duker JS, Puliafito CA. Indocyanine green angiography and choroidal neovascularization obscured by hemorrhage. *Ophthalmology.* 1995;102:1871-1876.

21. Flower RW, Csaky KG, Murphy RP. Disparity between fundus camera and scanning laser ophthalmoscope indocyanine green imaging of retinal pigment epithelium detachments. *Retina.* 1998;18:260-268.

22. Hope-Ross M, Yannuzzi LA, Gragoudas ES, et al. Adverse reactions due to indocyanine green. *Ophthalmology.* 1994;101:529-533.

23. Fernandes LH, Freund KB, Yannuzzi LA, et al. The nature of focal areas of hyperfluorescence or hot spots imaged with indocyanine green angiography. *Retina.* 2002;22:557-568.

24. Guyer DR, Yannuzzi LA, Slakter JS, et al. Classification of choroidal neovascularization by digital indocyanine green videoangiography. *Ophthalmology.* 1996;103:2054-2060.

25. Yannuzzi LA, Wong DW, Sforzolini BS, et al. Polypoidal choroidal vasculopathy and neovascularized age-related macular degeneration. *Arch Ophthalmol.* 1999;117:1503-1510.

26. Reichel E, Pollock DA, Duker JS, Puliafito CA. Indocyanine green angiography for recurrent choroidal neovascularization in age-related macular degeneration. *Ophthalmic Surg Lasers.* 1995;26(6):513-518.

27. Shiraga F, Ojima Y, Matsuo T, Takasu I, Matsuo N. Feeder vessel photocoagulation of subfoveal choroidal neovascularization secondary to age-related macular degeneration. *Ophthalmology.* 1998;105:662-669.

28. Staurenghi G, Orzalesi N, La Capria A, Aschero M. Laser treatment of feeder vessels in subfoveal choroidal neovascular membranes: a revisitation using dynamic indocyanine green angiography. *Ophthalmology.* 1998;105:2297-2305.

5

MIMICKERS OF AGE-RELATED MACULAR DEGENERATION

Kapil G. Kapoor, MD and Sophie J. Bakri, MD

Age-related macular degeneration (AMD) is the leading cause of severe visual impairment in the United States in individuals older than 65 years,[1,2] underscoring the importance of accurate diagnosis and treatment.[3] Although few effective treatment options existed for AMD in previous years, treatment options are now myriad and increasingly effective. This transition has further highlighted the importance of the accurate diagnosis of AMD. With the help of a variety of ophthalmic diagnostic imaging modalities and other clues in the patient's examination and history, a number of macular diseases can be differentiated from AMD. The differentiation of other disease entities from AMD often drastically affects patient treatment, follow-up, prognosis, and even psychology.[4] This chapter provides an approach for deciphering AMD from its potential mimickers.

It is helpful to categorize the mimickers of AMD into those imitating non-neovascular (dry) AMD and those imitating neovascular (wet) AMD, although these categories are not mutually exclusive. For the purposes of this chapter, these broad categories have been further divided into 3 subclassifications, each to facilitate a logical methodology to rapid and precise AMD diagnosis.

The classifications of dry AMD mimickers include:
- Macular dystrophies
- Drusen and its simulators
- Macular atrophy

The classifications of wet AMD mimickers include:
- Wet AMD variants
- Central serous retinopathy
- Choroidal neovascularization (CNV) and its simulators

Duker JS, Witkin AJ, eds.
Age-Related Macular Degeneration:
Current Management (pp. 75-92)
© 2015 Taylor & Francis Group

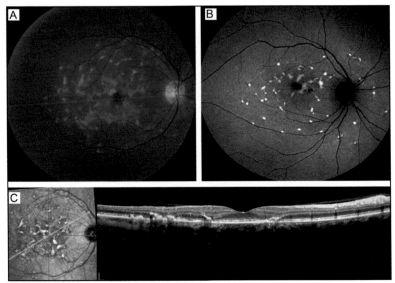

Figure 5-1. (A) Fundus photograph of the right eye in a patient with Stargardt's disease shows pisciform flecks at the level of the RPE. (B) FA better demonstrates the discrete boundaries of the pisciform flecks, which are hyperfluorescent here due to their lipofuscin composition. (C) OCT shows deposition of lipofuscin at the level of the RPE with localized patches of atrophy.

MIMICKERS OF DRY AGE-RELATED MACULAR DEGENERATION

Macular Dystrophies

Macular dystrophies represent an important cause of vision loss and are often included in the differential diagnosis of AMD. In contrast to AMD, the age of onset tends to be younger, and there is often a family history of a known diagnosis of vision loss at an early age. Between eyes, macular dystrophies typically exhibit striking symmetry. If the symmetry of the pattern is not initially evident on examination, fundus autofluorescence (FAF) often helps elucidate a more symmetric appearance because the dystrophies lead to typical patterns of lipofuscin accumulation in the macula. The most common macular dystrophies that may mimic AMD include Stargardt's disease (fundus flavimaculatus/juvenile macular dystrophy), Best's disease, and pattern dystrophies.[5]

Stargardt's disease is the most common inherited macular dystrophy.[6] It typically exhibits autosomal-recessive inheritance due to mutations in the ABCA4 gene, but it can also be associated with autosomal-dominant inheritance through the ELOVL4 gene mutation.[6,7] Phenotypically, Stargardt's disease is characterized by yellow, fish-shaped (or *pisciform*) flecks at the level of the retinal pigment epithelium (RPE) (Figure 5-1A). Piscifom flecks can be in the posterior pole but are often distributed throughout the fundus. When these flecks are distributed throughout the fundus, this is termed *fundus flavimaculatus*. These flecks often form reticular patterns that help distinguish them from drusen, although it can sometimes be difficult to distinguish the two clinically. FAF can better illustrate the discrete pisciform flecks because they are composed of lipofuscin, thus helping to distinguish the flecks from typical drusen that is associated with dry AMD (Figure 5-1B). Optical coherence tomography (OCT) of the flecks demonstrates accumulations of hyperreflective material at the level of the RPE (Figure 5-1C). Fluorescein angiography (FA) can demonstrate a dark choroid, which is a pathognomonic sign for the disease that is due to masked fluorescence of the choroid secondary to lipofuscin accumulation.[8] In its advanced stages, Stargardt's disease can resemble geographic atrophy secondary to AMD, and eliciting a family or personal history of visual deterioration beginning in the third decade may help to trigger genetic testing and accurate diagnosis.

Best's disease, or Best's vitelliform dystrophy, is characterized by the autosomal-dominant inheritance of a mutation in the VMD2 gene that encodes the protein bestrophin. It is classically characterized by a yellow, yolk-like macular lesion, associated with variable visual loss.[9,10] However, Best's disease progresses through a natural sequence of stages, many of which can mimic AMD. The previtelliform stage, which has subtle RPE changes, is followed by the vitelliform stage, which has a classic egg-yolk lesion. The pseudohypopyon stage comes next, involving layering of the lipofuscin and followed by breakup of this lipofuscin material in the vitelleruptive, or "scrambled egg," phase. The final stages involve atrophy and, in up to 20% of cases, CNV, both of which may be associated with significant visual loss. When clinical diagnosis is unclear, the electro-oculogram (EOG) will demonstrate an Arden ratio of 1.5 or less, whereas the electroretinogram (ERG) is typically normal; the abnormal EOG distinguishes this disease from AMD.[9,10] Genetic testing can also be pursued.

The pattern dystrophies are a group of heterogeneous, typically dominantly inherited conditions associated with unique macular patterns of lipofuscin deposition at the level of the RPE.[11] Pattern dystrophies can be confused with AMD, particularly in the earliest and advanced stages. In the early stages, pattern dystrophies often start with subtle RPE changes before evolving into a typical pattern; in advanced stages, they can progress to atrophy of the RPE (Figures 5-2A and B). FAF imaging can often help to delineate the symmetric phenotypic pattern of lipofuscin deposition that is typical of pattern dystrophy (Figures 5-2C and D). Genetic testing for the RDS/peripherin gene may also be helpful in making the diagnosis.

The patterns most typically encountered include the shape of a small egg yolk (adult-onset foveomacular vitelliform dystrophy), a butterfly (butterfly dystrophy), or a net (reticular dystrophies).[11-13] Adult-onset foveomacular vitelliform dystrophy is characterized by small, round, yellowish, subfoveal lesions that are bilateral and symmetric (Figures 5-3A and B). The patients with such a pattern can be distinguished from those with AMD by their typically earlier age of onset (30 to 50 years), striking symmetry on clinical examination, bilaterally circumscribed hyperfluorescence on FAF imaging (Figures 5-3C and D), and subretinal material deposition with inner segment/outer segment interface disruption noted on OCT (Figure 5-3E).[14,15] In patients with larger vitelliform lesions, a normal EOG can help to differentiate from Best's disease (Figure 5-3F). Butterfly dystrophy is associated with a triradiate pigment pattern resembling a butterfly (Figures 5-4A and B), which is more clearly elucidated by FAF imaging (Figures 5-4C and D). This can also be associated with increased peripheral pigment stippling.[12,14] Reticular dystrophy is associated with a fishnet pattern that denotes its reticular name. Management of pattern dystrophies typically consists of serial imaging

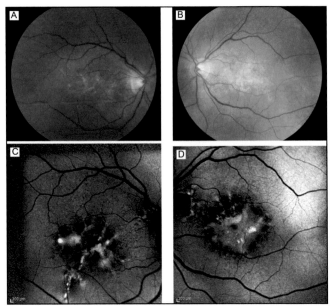

Figure 5-2. (A) Fundus photograph of a right eye demonstrates macular atrophy without drusen. (B) Fundus photograph of a left eye demonstrates symmetric macular atrophy without drusen. (C) FAF of a right eye delineates the symmetric pattern of lipofuscin deposition, which is typical of pattern dystrophy. (D) FAF of a left eye delineates the symmetric pattern of lipofuscin deposition, which is typical of pattern dystrophy.

with genetic testing, although up to 15% of patients may develop CNV, necessitating further intervention.[16]

Drusen and Its Simulators

Drusen in Diseases Other Than Age-Related Macular Degeneration

Drusen are yellowish, round, subretinal pigment epithelial deposits that are the hallmark of dry AMD; however, they can be seen in other conditions.[17] Familial drusen is a distinct cause of inherited macular drusen. Familial drusen has been classified into 4 different subtypes (although the distinction is mostly of historical interest): Hutchinson-Tay choroiditis, Holthouse-Batten chorioretinitis, Doyne's familial honeycombed choroiditis, and Malattia leventinese.[18] Familial drusen typically has an autosomal-dominant inheritance pattern (and is therefore sometimes referred to as *dominant drusen*), although other inheritance patterns have also been described.[19] Both Malattia leventinese and Doyne's familial honeycombed choroiditis have a mutation in the gene coding for an epidermal growth factor containing a fibulin-like extracellular matrix protein (EFEMP1).[19,20] These patients tend to present earlier in age (third to fifth decade) than AMD and often have a family history. Their drusen are also distinct because they tend to form in an elongated, radiating pattern, frequently extending beyond the arcades, particularly nasally.[20]

Important causes of midperipheral drusen also exist, such as membranoproliferative glomerulonephritis (types 1 and 2), and Alport's syndrome.[21] These entities can be

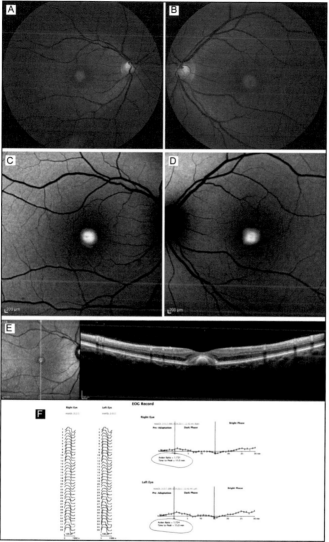

Figure 5-3. (A) Fundus photograph of a right eye demonstrates subfoveal vitelliform material with central pigment clumping, which is typical of adult-onset foveomacular vitelliform dystrophy. (B) Fundus photograph of a left eye demonstrates subfoveal vitelliform material with central pigment clumping, which is typical of adult-onset foveomacular vitelliform dystrophy. (C) FAF of a right eye demonstrates hyperfluorescence of vitelliform material, confirming its lipofuscin composition. (D) FAF of a left eye demonstrates hyperfluorescence of vitelliform material, confirming its lipofuscin composition. (E) OCT demonstrates subfoveal deposition of subretinal material. (F) EOG testing reveals a normal Arden ratio of 1.73 in the right eye and 1.72 in the left eye, ruling out Best's disease and confirming the diagnosis of adult-onset foveomacular vitelliform dystrophy.

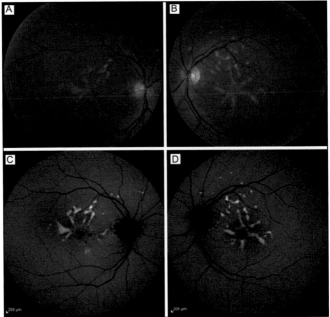

Figure 5-4. (A) Fundus photograph of a right eye shows a radiate, butterfly-pattern dystrophy. (B) Fundus photograph of a left eye shows a radiate, butterfly-pattern dystrophy. (C) FAF of a right eye shows hyperfluorescence of a lipofuscin deposition pattern, consistent with butterfly-pattern dystrophy. (D) FAF of a left eye shows hyperfluorescence of a lipofuscin deposition pattern, consistent with butterfly-pattern dystrophy.

distinguished from AMD because they tend to present earlier in age. Although they can concentrate in the posterior pole, extensive drusen throughout the midperiphery beyond the arcades is also typical (Figures 5-5A and B). Alport's syndrome can also be associated with anterior lenticonus (Figure 5-5C). An association with CNV has been described, further underscoring the importance of eliciting a history of renal problems when this distribution of drusen is noted.[22]

Crystalline Deposits

Crystalline deposits in the retina can simulate calcified macular drusen, sometimes posing a particular diagnostic challenge because both can form in the posterior pole and may have a refractile appearance.

Macular telangiectasia type 2 (MacTel 2) is a condition that is associated with crystals and is commonly confused with wet AMD; therefore, it is discussed in more detail in the next section of this chapter.[23]

Bietti crystalline dystrophy is characterized by an autosomal-recessive inheritance pattern, with initial patches of localized atrophy often progressing to coalesced patterns of atrophy. It can be distinguished from AMD because crystal deposition can occur in both the retina and the cornea, and it typically begins at an earlier age (third to fifth decade).[24]

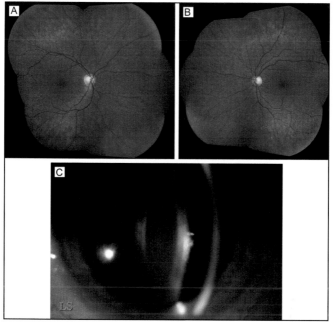

Figure 5-5. (A) Fundus photograph of the right eye of a patient with Alport's syndrome shows symmetric dense midperipheral drusen. (B) Fundus photograph of the left eye of a patient with Alport's syndrome shows symmetric dense midperipheral drusen. (C) Anterior segment photograph shows mild anterior lenticonus in a patient with Alport's syndrome.

Crystalline deposits in the retina can also be associated with drug toxicity, including intravenous methadone or meperidine (demonstrated as talc retinopathy), tamoxifen (antineoplastic agent), methoxyflurane (anesthetic), and canthaxanthine (oral tanning agent).[25] Eliciting a detailed history can help to distinguish these etiologies from AMD.

Systemic conditions have also been described with crystalline retinal deposits, including oxalosis, cystinosis, hyperornithinemia, and Sjögren-Larsson syndrome.[25] Patients with oxalosis have diffuse deposition of calcium oxalate in various tissues of the body, and a history of nephrolithiasis is often present.[26] Hyperornithinemia is associated with progressive gyrate atrophy throughout the fundus, and it can have colorless, elongated, glittering crystalline deposits.[27] Cystinosis is a rare autosomal-recessive lysosomal storage disorder that is also associated with diffuse crystalline deposition, and it is typically associated with severe renal dysfunction, necessitating renal transplant in the first decade of life.[28] Sjögren-Larsson syndrome is a rare autosomal-recessive disease associated with perifoveal yellowish-white crystals in the first decade of life.[25] It is typically associated with congenital ichthyosis, spasticity, and mental retardation. A complete review of systems with multidisciplinary health evaluation can be important in patients with crystalline deposition to rule out systemic causes.

Flecks

Macular pathologies assuming a punctuate distribution of yellowish or whitish flecks can also imitate drusen and be confused for AMD. A heterogeneous group of disorders causing flecks in the retina can simulate this appearance.

Benign familial flecked retina is one such condition that is associated with autosomal-recessive inheritance. It typically presents with flecks of discrete, yellowish-white, polymorphous shapes that are diffusely present in the fundus, extending to the far periphery. This is distinguished from AMD by its diffuse distribution that spares the fovea and maintenance of excellent visual acuity. Fundus albipunctatus is a separate condition that can have a similar fundus appearance, but it is associated with nyctalopia and an abnormal ERG.[29] Fleck retina of Kandori is a rare condition that is characterized by irregular, sharply defined, yellowish, large flecks of the retina and is associated with nyctalopia.[30] Careful ophthalmoscopy can help to distinguish these flecked conditions from AMD, but family history and ERG can be useful tools to aid in the diagnosis.

Macular Atrophy

Bull's Eye Maculopathy

Bull's eye maculopathy refers to the specific pattern of foveal hyperpigmentation surrounded by a zone of depigmentation, which is in turn surrounded by an annulus of hyperpigmentation. This pattern of atrophy is classically associated with hydroxychloroquine toxicity, but it can also be associated with the following[31]:

- Stargardt's disease
- Cone dystrophy
- Cone-rod dystrophy
- Autoimmune retinopathy
- Central areolar choroidal atrophy
- Fenestrated sheen macular dystrophy
- Olivopontocerebellar atrophy
- Ceroid lipofuscinosis

In some cases, geographic atrophy (GA) in AMD can coalesce to an annular pattern, sparing a central foveal island and bearing a striking resemblance to bull's eye maculopathy. Typically, the causes of bull's eye maculopathy can be distinguished from AMD because AMD occurs later in life, has associated drusen, and often has a multifocal pattern of geographic atrophy that coalesces. Family history and further testing through genetics, FAF, and ERG can prove useful in diagnosis (Figure 5-6).

Other Causes of Macular Atrophy

Myopic degeneration is another important cause of macular atrophy that can mimic AMD. Important distinguishing features of myopic degeneration include a history of refractive error that is consistent with high myopia (more than −6.00 diopters or an axial length greater than 26.5 mm)[32] and a tigroid or tessellated fundus appearance secondary to diffuse attenuation of the RPE, with visibility of the choroidal vasculature. Examination can also reveal tilted discs, peripapillary atrophy, lacquer cracks, Forster-Fuchs spots, or a staphyloma, in addition to the notable absence of drusen and often younger age of onset.[32,33]

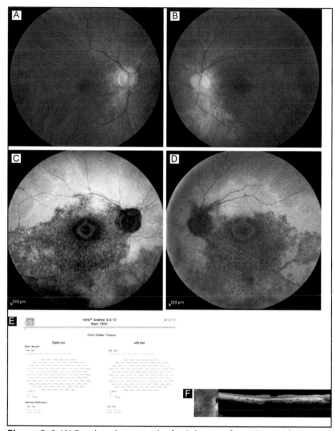

Figure 5-6. (A) Fundus photograph of a right eye of a patient with autoimmune retinopathy shows hyperpigmentation surrounded by an annulus of hypopigmentation, consistent with bull's eye maculopathy. (B) Fundus photograph of the left eye of a patient with autoimmune retinopathy shows hyperpigmentation surrounded by an annulus of hypopigmentation, consistent with bull's eye maculopathy. (C) FAF of a right eye shows stippled hypofluorescence radiating from a central bull's eye pattern, suggesting diffuse dysfunction of the RPE. (D) FAF of a left eye shows stippled hypofluorescence radiating from a central bull's eye pattern, suggesting diffuse dysfunction of the RPE. (E) Multifocal ERG shows flat waveforms consistent with diffuse macular dysfunction. (F) OCT delineates RPE atrophy sparing a central foveal island.

North Carolina macular dystrophy is a rare autosomal-dominant form of inherited macular degeneration that often progresses to bilateral symmetric macular atrophy early in life. The genetic location has been identified (MCDR1) on chromosome 6q14-q16.2; however, no causative gene has yet been identified. In the early stages of North Carolina macular dystrophy, only drusen are evident, but this can progress to RPE atrophy and eventually to GA. Often, visual acuity is better than one would expect with the degree of atrophy present.[34]

Any condition associated with CNV can be associated with variable macular atrophy and scarring, in turn mimicking AMD. These will be discussed in detail in the next section.

MIMICKERS OF WET AGE-RELATED MACULAR DEGENERATION

Wet Age-Related Macular Degeneration Variants

Traditional classifications of wet AMD define the subtypes of CNV as *classic* and *occult* (as discussed in Chapter 4). Evolving diagnostic technology, particularly spectral-domain OCT and indocyanine green angiography (ICG), has demonstrated that the spectrum of wet AMD is more complex than previously understood. Important variants of wet AMD include retinal angiomatous proliferation (RAP) and polypoidal choroidal vasculopathy (PCV).

RAP is a variant of wet AMD that is characterized by the formation of pathologic new vessels within the retina that secondarily invade the subretinal space or choroid.[35] This has also been termed type 3 neovascularization and has been estimated to account for approximately 15% of cases of wet AMD.[35] RAP evolves through an initial stage of intra-retinal neovascularization with telangiectatic retinal capillaries (stage I), followed by extension into the subretinal space, with associated subretinal neovascularization and a serous RPE detachment (stage II), eventually progressing to a complete retinal-choroidal anastomosis (stage III) (Figure 5-7).[36]

PCV is a disease that likely comes in 2 varieties: a distinct disease from AMD (typically found in a younger age group than AMD, without other fundus findings typical of AMD) and as a subset of wet AMD. PCV is characterized by a branching network of polyp-like vessels, often having an increased tendency to form exudation and subretinal hemorrhage.[37] PCV tends to occur in the peripapillary region, with increased incidence in Asian individuals. Indocyanine green angiography (ICGA) is the best tool to visualize the vessels, and it is an important consideration to pursue in patients diagnosed with wet AMD who are refractory to treatment (Figure 5-8).

Central Serous Retinopathy

Central serous chorioretinopathy (CSC) is an important mimicker of AMD. It typically presents in men in the fourth to sixth decade of life, with a potential association with type-A personality and corticosteroid administration. Examination and OCT testing can reveal subretinal fluid and RPE detachments out of proportion to intraretinal findings (Figures 5-9A-D) Enhanced-depth imaging OCT often reveals increased choroidal thickness (see Chapter 4, Section 2).[38] FA can reveal patterns of leakage, such as an expansile dot, a smokestack, or a diffuse pattern of hyperfluorescence. ICGA is often useful because it may demonstrate a pattern of choroidal vascular hyperpermeability (Figures 5-9E-F).[38] Treatment of CSC may be performed with focal laser or photodynamic therapy after a variable period of observation. Other systemic oral medications have also been tried with variable success. Because this treatment paradigm clearly deviates from that of wet AMD, it further underscores the importance of differentiating this important AMD mimicker to optimize patient outcomes.

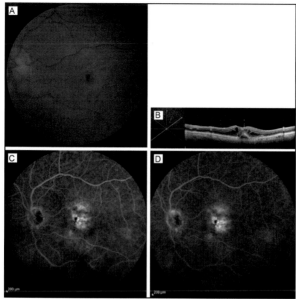

Figure 5-7. (A) Fundus photograph of a left eye shows foveal intraretinal hemorrhage with surrounding cystoid macular edema from a retinal angiomatous proliferative lesion. (B) OCT of a left eye shows a pigment epithelial detachment with overlying intraretinal fluid. (C) FA (early) reveals blockage from intraretinal hemorrhage with perifoveal petalloid leakage, which is consistent with cystoid macular edema. (D) FA (late) reveals blockage from intraretinal hemorrhage and confirms late leakage, which is consistent with cystoid macular edema.

Macular Telangiectasia

MacTel (types 1 and 2) is a condition that can be confused with wet AMD. In addition to being associated with crystals, as discussed previously, MacTel can also be associated with secondary subretinal neovascular membranes that can mimic the appearance of CNV seen in wet AMD. Previously known as *idiopathic juxtafoveal telangiectasia*, it occurs in 2 main subtypes. Type 1 is typically unilateral, predominantly in males, and associated with aneurysms and exudates. It is likely a mild "form fruste" variant of Coats' disease. OCT of type 1 MacTel typically demonstrates macular edema as well as hyper-reflective hard exudates. Type 2 is more common than type 1, is typically bilateral, and affects both sexes equally. Other types of MacTel have also been described (such as type 3, associated with bilateral occlusive telangiectasias), but these are much more rare and are likely subtypes of types 1 and 2.[23] Because type 2 is the most common, this is typically what is referred to as MacTel, and it is the type most commonly discussed in the literature.

Key distinguishing features of MacTel 2 from AMD include the bilateral and symmetric location of telangiectatic vessels just temporal to the fovea, sometimes associated with pigment clumping and right-angle venules. These patients are also younger than AMD patients, presenting around the fifth decade, and often a history of diabetes mellitus can be

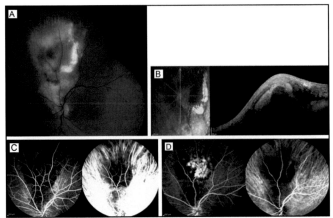

Figure 5-8. (A) Fundus photograph montage of a left eye shows peripapillary subretinal hemorrhage, subretinal fluid, and exudation from an active polypoidal choroidal vasculopathy network. (B) OCT through this region demonstrates subretinal hemorrhage, subretinal fluid, and exudates. (C) FA (left panel) and ICGA (right panel) of the left eye (early) show peripapillary polyp-like vessels, consistent with PCV. (D) FA (left panel) and ICGA (right panel) of the left eye (late) show leakage from polyp-like vessels, consistent with active PCV.

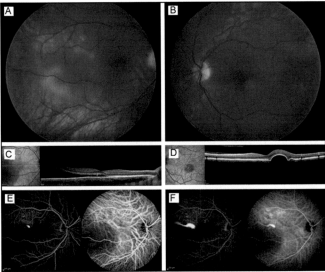

Figure 5-9. (A) Fundus photograph right eye shows subretinal fluid temporal to the fovea in a patient with active CSR. (B) Fundus photograph of a left eye shows pigment epithelial detachment with pigment clumping, consistent with chronic CSR. (C) OCT of a right eye confirms significant subretinal fluid. (D) OCT of a left eye shows serous pigment epithelial detachment. (F) FA (left panel) and ICGA (right panel) of a right eye (early) show focal area of hyperfluorescence just temporal to the fovea. (F) FA (left panel) and ICGA (right panel) of a right eye (late) show leakage from area of choroidal hyperpermeability, consistent with CSR.

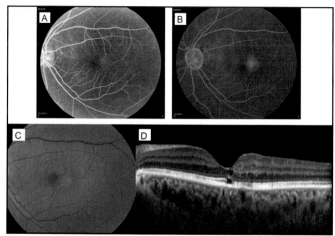

Figure 5-10. (A) Early FA of the left eye shows telangiectatic vessels in the temporal macula. (B) Late FA of the left eye shows leakage from these telagiectatic vessels. (C) Fundus photograph left eye shows a whitish sheen in the region of telagiectatic vessels, due to tiny crystalline lesions in the temporal macula. (D) OCT reveals a normal inner retinal contour, outer retinal (photoreceptor) disruption, and small intraretinal cystic spaces representing loss of foveal tissue, with a thin "ILM drape" covering the roof of the cystic space.

elicited. OCT testing typically reveals a normal inner retinal contour, outer retinal (photoreceptor) disruption, and small intraretinal cystic spaces representing loss of foveal tissue, often with a thin internal limiting membrane drape covering the roof of the cystic space. FA can help elucidate the telangiectatic vessels and distinguish MacTel 2 from AMD.[23]

Causes of Choroidal Neovascularization Other Than AMD

CNV is most frequently encountered in wet AMD, but it can stem from multiple other etiologies that destabilize Bruch's membrane or damage the RPE. These include infectious uveitis such as toxoplasmosis (Figure 5-10); noninfectious uveitis such as the white-dot syndromes (Figure 5-11); peripapillary pathology such as angioid streaks or optic disc drusen; macular dystrophies such as Sorsby's (a rare autosomal-dominant cause of bilateral CNV, due to a defect in the gene encoding TIMP-3)[39]; choroidal tumors such as nevus, melanoma, and osteoma (Figure 5-12); degenerative conditions such as myopia; iatrogenic conditions such as prior laser treatments; trauma such as choroidal rupture; presumed ocular histoplasmosis; or idiopathic causes.[40-42] Often, these conditions lead to CNV that appears classic on FA, and they often respond well to anti-VEGF therapies. Detailed history, ocular examination, and imaging can help aid in diagnosis.

Pathologic myopia is one of the most common causes of non-AMD–related CNV. Myopia can lead to lacquer cracks, which are disruptions in Bruch's membrane. These cracks are a pathway for CNV lesions to grow through and underneath the retina. Angioid streaks are typically bilateral, linear, thin breaks in Bruch's membrane that emanate from the optic disc and may give the appearance of deep vessels (hence the term *angioid*). These may be associated with a variety of connective tissue disorders, particularly pseudoxanthoma elasticum, but can be idiopathic in nature.[41,42]

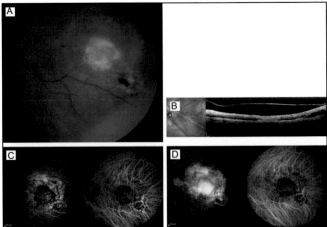

Figure 5-11. Fundus photograph of a left eye shows a yellowish scar inferotemporal to the fovea with surrounding intraretinal fluid and vitreomacular traction in a patient with a history of toxoplasma retinochoroiditis and secondary CNV. (B) OCT of a left eye confirms scarring inferotemporal to the fovea with surrounding intraretinal fluid and vitreomacular traction. (C) FA (left panel) and ICGA (right panel) (early) show hyperfluorescence of toxoplasmosis scarring with no activity on ICGA, suggesting no reactivation of the CNV. (D) FA (left panel) and ICGA (right panel) (late) show leakage consistent with reactivation of toxoplasmosis retinochoroiditis, with no activity on ICGA, suggesting no reactivation of CNV.

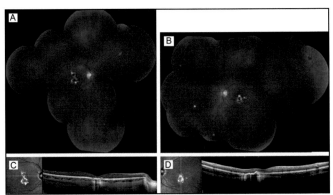

Figure 5-12. (A) Fundus montage of a right eye shows macular scarring and few peripheral scars in a patient with multifocal choroiditis and a history of secondary CNV. (B) Fundus montage of a left eye showing macular scarring and few peripheral scars in a patient with multifocal choroiditis and a history of secondary CNV. (C) OCT confirms atrophy with the absence of intraretinal or subretinal fluid, suggesting CNV is inactive. (D) OCT confirms atrophy with absence of intraretinal or subretinal fluid, suggesting CNV is inactive.

Choroidal inflammatory disorders can cause CNV lesions to form both during active disease (eg, multifocal choroiditis) or after they have caused a macular scar to form (eg, presumed ocular histoplasmosis syndrome), creating a disruption in Bruch's membrane

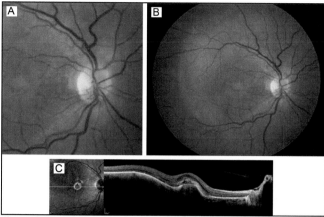

Figure 5-13. (A) Macular photograph of a right eye shows a greenish, coin-shaped lesion consistent with CNV in the fovea. (B) Fundus photograph of a right eye reveals malignant uveal melanoma along the superotemporal arcade associated with previously noted CNV. (C) OCT demonstrates temporal choroidal thickening from choroidal melanoma with foveal CNV and associated overlying intraretinal fluid.

and a nidus for a CNV lesion to grow.[40] Presumed ocular histoplasmosis syndrome (POHS) is of particular interest in the United States because the Ohio and Mississippi River valleys are endemic to the organism *Histoplasma capsulatum*, and a high incidence of adults in these regions have eye findings consistent with POHS. Findings suggestive of POHS include a triad of atrophic discreet chorioretinal lesions, peripapillary scarring, and a CNV membrane.[42]

Other Causes of Macular Hemorrhage

Posterior pole lesions can present with macular hemorrhages in the preretinal, intraretinal, subretinal, and/or sub-RPE space, and although it is often tempting to suggest CNV as the source, it remains important to consider the other causes in this broad differential. A ruptured macroaneurysm can be a source of macular hemorrhage, classically presenting with hemorrhage in 3 layers (pre-, intra-, and subretinal) (Figure 5-13). The density of the patient's blood can make identifying the source difficult, but examination may reveal a white center of the ruptured macroaneurysm, and FA can reveal a hyperfluorescent saccular outpouching along a retinal arterial vessel, coinciding with the ruptured macroaneurysm. A history of hypertension and diabetes, often with changes of hypertensive retinopathy in the contralateral eye, can further aid in diagnosis (Figure 5-14).[43]

Valsalva retinopathy can be associated with macular hemorrhages, which can be sub-, intra-, or preretinal in nature, and with a history of coughing, straining, or other strenuous activity as a source of valsalva.[44] Posterior pole tumors, such as choroidal melanoma, can rarely be associated with breakthrough bleeding from the choroid into the subretinal space or vitreous cavity. Ultrasound can prove useful in demonstrating choroidal thickness from a tumor when fundus examination prohibits a detailed view. Proliferative diabetic retinopathy is an important source of macular hemorrhages, but these typically are preretinal in location, particularly in the subhyaloid space. A history of diabetes

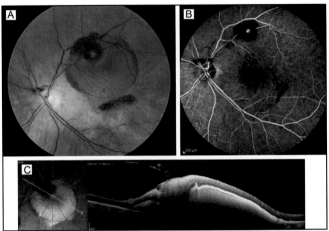

Figure 5-14. (A) Fundus photograph of a left eye reveals a massive subretinal macular hemorrhage with associated preretinal hemorrhage. (B) FA of a left eye shows hyperfluorescence from saccular outpouching along the superotemporal arcade, confirming a ruptured macroaneurysm as the etiology of the subretinal hemorrhage. (C) OCT through a lesion demonstrates that it is predominantly subretinal, with a component of intraretinal hemorrhage and associated breakthrough bleeding into the vitreous cavity.

mellitus with diabetic retinopathy evident in both eyes and fronds of neovascularization demonstrated on examination or by FA aid in the diagnosis.

SUMMARY

With the influx of effective treatment strategies for AMD, it is increasingly important to accurately diagnose AMD. This chapter has attempted to lay a foundation through diagnostic clues to deciphering AMD from mimickers of both its dry and wet forms. Increasing awareness of conditions that mimic AMD will increase clinician effectiveness and ultimately optimize patient outcomes.

REFERENCES

1. Klein R, Lee KE, Gangnon RE, Klein BE. Incidence of visual impairment over a 20-year period: the Beaver Dam Eye Study. *Ophthalmology*. 2013;130(6):1210-1219.
2. Klein R, Klein BEK, Linton KLP. Prevalence of age-related maculopathy: the Beaver Dam Eye Study. *Ophthalmology*. 1992;99:933-943.
3. Current population reports population projections of the United States by age, sex, race, and hispanic origin: 1995-2050. Washington, DC: United States Bureau of the Census; 1996. Series P25-P1130.
4. Bennion AE, Shaw RL, Gibson JM. What do we know about the experience of age-related macular degeneration? A systematic review and meta-synthesis of qualitative research. *Soc Sci Med*. 2012;75(6):976-985.
5. Dosunmu EO, Bakri SJ. Mimickers of age-related macular degeneration. *Semin Ophthalmol*. 2011;26(3):209-215.
6. Noemi L, Holder GE, Bunce C, et al. Phenotypic subtypes of Stargardt macular dystrophy-fundus flavimaculatus. *Arch Ophthalmol*. 2001;119:359-369.

7. Westerfeld C, Mukai S. Stargardt's disease and the ABCR gene. *Semin Ophthalmol.* 2008;23(1):59-65.

8. Fishman GA. Inherited macular dystrophies: a clinical overview. *Aust N Z J Ophthalmol.* 1990;18(2):123-128.

9. Krill AE, Morse PA, Potts AM, Klien BA. Hereditary vitelliruptive macular degeneration. *Am J Ophthalmol.* 1966;61(6):1405-1415.

10. Kobrin JL, Apple DJ, Hart WB. Vitelliform dystrophy. *Int Ophthalmol Clin.* 1981;21(3):167-184.

11. Hsieh RC, Fine BS, Lyons JS. Patterned dystrophies of the retinal pigment epithelium. *Arch Ophthalmol.* 1977;95(3):429-435.

12. Deutman AF, van Blommestein JD, Henkes HE, et al. Butterfly-shaped pigment dystrophy of the fovea. *Arch Ophthalmol.* 1970;83:558-569.

13. Gass JD. A clinicopathologic study of a peculiar foveomacular dystrophy. *Trans Am Ophthalmol Soc.* 1974;72:139-156.

14. Kingham JD, Fenzl RE, Willerson D, Aaberg TM. Reticular dystrophy of the retinal pigment epithelium: a clinical and electrophysiologic study of three generations. *Arch Ophthalmol.* 1978;96(7):1177-1184.

15. Fishman GA, Trimble S, Rabb MF, Fishman M. Pseudovitelliform macular degeneration. *Arch Ophthalmol.* 1977;95(1):73-76.

16. Francis PJ, Schultz DW, Gregory AM, et al. Genetic and phenotypic heterogeneity in pattern dystrophy. *Br J Ophthalmol.* 2005;89:1115-1119.

17. Abdelsalam A, Del Priore L, Zarbin MA. Drusen in age-related macular degeneration: pathogenesis, natural course, and laser photocoagulation-induced regression. *Surv Ophthalmol.* 1999;44(1):1-29.

18. Piguet B, Haimovici R, Bird AC. Dominantly inherited drusen represent more than one disorder: a historical review. *Eye (Lond).* 1995;9:34-41.

19. Deutman AF, Jansen LM. Dominantly inherited drusen of Bruch's membrane. *Br J Ophthalmol.* 1970;54:373-382.

20. Heon E, Piguet B, Munier F, et al. Linkage of autosomal dominant radial drusen (malattia leventinese) to chromosome 2p16-21. *Arch Ophthalmol.* 1996;114(2):193-198.

21. Han DP, Sievers S. Extensive drusen in type I membranoproliferative glomerulonephritis. *Arch Ophthalmol.* 2009;127(4):577-579.

22. Hassenstein A, Gisbert R. Choroidal neovascularization in type II membranoproliferative glomerulonephritis, photodynamic therapy as a treatment option: a case report. *Klin Montasbl Augenheilkd.* 2003;220(7):492-495.

23. Yannuzzi LA, Bardal AM, Freund KB, Chen KJ, Eandi CM, Blodi B. Idiopathic macular telangiectasias. *Arch Ophthalmol.* 2006;124:450-460.

24. Welch RB. Bietti's tapetoretinal degeneration with marginal corneal dystrophy crystalline retinopathy. *Trans Am Ophthalmol Soc.* 1977;75:164-179.

25. Nadim F, Walid H, Adib J. The differential diagnosis of crystals in the retina. *Int Ophthalmol.* 2002;24:113-121.

26. Farrel J, Shoemaker JD, Otti T, et al. Primary hyperoxaluria in an adult with renal failure, livedo reticularis, retinopathy and peripheral neuropathy. *Am J Kidney Dis.* 1997;29:947-952.

27. Bhaduri G. Gyrate atrophy of the choroid and retina. *J Indian Med Assoc.* 2002;100(3):196-197.

28. Town M, Jean G, Cherqui S, et al. A novel gene encoding an integral membrane protein is mutated in nephropathic cystinosis. *Nat Genet.* 1998;18(4):319-324.

29. Marmor F. Long-term follow-up of the physiologic abnormalities and fundus changes in fundus albipunctatus. *Ophthalmology.* 1990;97(3):380-384.

30. Kandori F. Very rare cases of congenital non-progressive nightblindness with fleck retina. *Jpn J Ophthalmol.* 1959;13:394.

31. Kurz-Levin MM, Halfyard AS, Bunce C, Bird AC, Holder GE. Clinical variations in assessment of bull's-eye maculopathy. *Arch Ophthalmol.* 2002;120(5):567-575.

32. Miller DG, Singerman LJ. Natural history of choroidal neovascularization in high myopia. *Curr Opin Ophthalmol.* 2001;12(3):222-224.

33. Hayashi K, Ohno-Matsui K, Shimada N, et al. Long-term pattern of progression of myopic maculopathy: a natural history study. *Ophthalmology*. 2010;117(8):1595-1611.

34. Khurana RN, Sun X, Pearson E, et al. A reappraisal of the clinical spectrum of North Carolina macular dystrophy. *Ophthalmology*. 2009;116(10):1976-1983.

35. Yannuzzi LA, Negrao S, Iida T, et al. Retinal angiomatous proliferation in age-related macular degeneration. *Retina*. 2001;21:416-434.

36. Freund KB, Ho IV, Barbazetto IA, et al. Type 3 neovascularization: the expanded spectrum of retinal angiomatous proliferation. *Retina*. 2008;28:201-211.

37. Lim TH, Laude A, Tan CS. Polypoidal choroidal vasculopathy: an angiographic discussion. *Eye (Lond)*. 2010;24:483-490.

38. Nicholson B, Noble J, Forooghian F, Meyerle C. Central serous chorioretinopathy: update on pathophysiology and treatment. *Surv Ophthalmol*. 2013;58(2):103-126.

39. Weber BH, Vogt G, Pruett RC, Stohr H, Felbor U. Mutations in the tissue inhibitor of metalloproteinases-3 (TIMP3) in patients with Sorsby's fundus dystrophy. *Nat Genet*. 1994;8:352-356.

40. Neri P, Lettieri M, Fortuna C, Manoni M, Giovannini A. Inflammatory choroidal neovascularization. *Middle East Afr J Ophthalmol*. 2009;16(4):245-251.

41. Cohen SY, Laroche A, Leguen Y, Soubrane G, Coscas GJ. Etiology of choroidal neovascularization in young patients. *Ophthalmology*. 1996;103(8):1241-1244.

42. Spaide RF. Choroidal neovascularization in younger patients. *Curr Opin Ophthalmol*. 1999;10(3):177-181.

43. McCabe CM, Flynn HW Jr, McLean WC, et al. Nonsurgical management of macular hemorrhage secondary to retinal artery macroaneurysms. *Arch Ophthalmol*. 2000;118:780-786.

44. Lavezzo MM, Zacharias LC, Takahashi WY. Sub-internal limiting membrane hemorrhage in Valsalva retinopathy: case report. *Arq Bras Oftalmol*. 2012;75(6):436-438.

6

INTRAVITREAL ANTI-VASCULAR ENDOTHELIAL GROWTH FACTOR THERAPY

Mariana R. Thorell, MD and Philip J. Rosenfeld, MD, PhD

Vascular endothelial growth factor A (VEGF-A) is the major angiogenic and vascular permeability factor implicated in the pathogenesis of many retinal vascular diseases, including neovascular (wet) age-related macular degeneration (AMD).[1] Four major isoforms of VEGF-A have been identified in humans ($VEGF_{121}$, $VEGF_{165}$, $VEGF_{189}$, and $VEGF_{206}$), and at least 5 minor isoforms are known ($VEGF_{145}$, $VEGF_{148}$, $VEGF_{162}$, $VEGF_{165b}$, and $VEGF_{183}$).[2,3] The nomenclature used to designate the different isoforms refers to the number of amino acids that compose the secreted protein[4]; the most prevalent form is $VEGF_{165}$.[5] The association between pathologic neovascularization in the eye and the expression of VEGF-A is unambiguous and suggests that local inhibition of VEGF-A can be a strategy for the treatment of neovascular eye disease.[4,6-8]

The introduction of therapies using inhibitors of VEGF has revolutionized the treatment of wet AMD, resulting in significant improvements in visual acuity. The objective of treatment with intravitreal anti-VEGF injections is to eliminate leakage of fluid and/or blood in the macula and prevent or slow the growth of choroidal neovascularization (CNV). The decision to treat or not to treat can be based on the presence of macular fluid seen on optical coherence tomography (OCT) images, as discussed in Chapter 5. Four anti-VEGF agents have been used clinically for the treatment of wet AMD: pegaptanib sodium (Macugen; OSI/Eyetech), bevacizumab (Avastin; Genentech), ranibizumab (Lucentis; Genentech), aflibercept (Eylea; Regeneron).

Randomized clinical trials were essential in determining the acceptance of these anti-VEGF therapies as first-line treatments for wet AMD, although anecdotal reports of the success of bevacizumab therapy led to it becoming widely used prior to results from a randomized clinical trial (as discussed later). Pegapatanib sodium is now essentially obsolete for the treatment of wet AMD.[9-13] Currently, intravitreal bevacizumab, ranibizumab, and aflibercept are the 3 medications commonly used to treat wet AMD in clinical practice, and these drugs produce significant improvements in the retinal anatomy and in visual outcomes when compared with other therapies.[14-16]

Duker JS, Witkin AJ, eds.
Age-Related Macular Degeneration:
Current Management (pp. 93-109)
© 2015 Taylor & Francis Group

PEGAPTANIB SODIUM

Pegaptanib sodium is an RNA aptamer that has high affinity and specificity to bind to human $VEGF_{165}$. The drug was the first VEGF-A inhibitor approved by the US Food and Drug Administration (FDA) for the treatment of wet AMD in 2004 based on 2 phase II/III multicenter, randomized, double-masked, sham-controlled, 2-year studies, known as the VEGF Inhibition Study in Ocular Neovascularization (VISION). In these clinical trials, patients with wet AMD were randomly assigned to receive intravitreal injections of pegaptanib sodium (doses of 0.3, 1.0, or 3.0 mg) or sham injections every 6 weeks for 48 weeks. Patients with predominantly classic lesions could receive photodynamic therapy at baseline and during the study at the discretion of the investigator. At week 54, the pegaptanib group was re-randomized (1:1) to continue or discontinue therapy for a period of 48 more weeks. Patients in the sham group were also re-randomized (1:1:1:1:1) and could continue with sham injections, discontinue sham injections, or receive one of the 3 doses of pegaptanib sodium.[17-20] One-year results demonstrated that all 3 doses of pegaptanib were effective in preventing vision loss when compared with sham injection, although there was a mean loss of visual acuity in all groups.[6,21] At 2 years, the proportion of patients that lost visual acuity was lower in the 0.3-mg pegaptanib group that continued treatment for 2 years than in the group that initially was treated with 0.3 mg of pegaptanib but then discontinued treatment after 1 year.[17,19]

Pegaptanib was approved in December 2004 and became commercially available in January 2005; however, its clinical use was soon supplanted by bevacizumab in 2005. The use of pegaptanib sodium has now become of historical interest only because the other anti-VEGF agents discussed in this chapter have been shown to be far superior in efficacy.

BEVACIZUMAB

Bevacizumab is a full-length monoclonal antibody that binds all biologically active isoforms of VEGF-A.[16,22] This drug was approved by the FDA in 2004 as an intravenous treatment for metastatic colorectal cancer.[22-24] As a treatment for wet AMD, intravenous bevacizumab was first used with remarkable benefit in a prospective pilot study known as the Systemic Bevacizumab (Avastin) therapy for Neovascular AMD.[25] However, due to the increased risk of thromboembolic events from the high dose of systemic bevacizumab, intravenous treatment was not ideal.

Around the same time, the same authors performed the first intravitreal injection of bevacizumab in a patient with wet AMD, showing dramatic improvement on OCT and in visual acuity, similar to the results from the intravenous bevacizumab study.[26] Soon after, several studies reported significant improvement in mean visual acuity and reduced OCT central retinal thickness in patients with wet AMD using intravitreal bevacizumab at doses ranging from 1.25 to 2.5 mg,[27-40] and off-label use of low-dose intravitreal bevacizumab became popular worldwide for the treatment of wet AMD. Notably, several studies showed good response to the medication, but there was no evidence from a large randomized clinical trial regarding the use of bevacizumab for wet AMD until the Comparision of Age-Related Macular Degeneration Treatment Trial (CATT) results were released in 2012.

Recently, some concern has emerged regarding potential contamination issues when using intravitreal bevacizumab. Because bevacizumab is only formulated for nonocular use in 4- and 16-mL vials, it must be aliquoted by a compounding pharmacy into individual intravitreal doses for off-label treatment of wet AMD. Non-standardization in compounding techniques has led to a few outbreaks of endophthalmitis around the world; therefore, care should be taken by each physician prescribing intravitreal bevacizumab to ensure that the compounding pharmacy uses proper sterilization techniques. In the United States, most experts have agreed that compounding pharmacies should adhere to the principles set forth in the United States Pharmacopeia chapter 797, which provides widely accepted national standards and guidelines for sterile preparations.[41]

RANIBIZUMAB

Ranibizumab is a recombinant, humanized, monoclonal antibody antigen-binding fragment that binds and inhibits all known active forms of VEGF-A.[42,43] Both bevacizumab and ranibizumab are derived from the same murine monoclonal antibody against VEGF and bind to the same epitope on VEGF. Ranibizumab was FDA approved in June 2006 based on 2 important phase III trials: MARINA (Minimally Classic/Occult Trial of the Anti-VEGF Antibody Ranibizumab in the Treatment of Neovascular AMD) and ANCHOR (Anti-VEGF Antibody Ranibizumab for the Treatment of Predominantly Classic Choroidal Neovascularization in AMD). These pivotal studies used monthly injections of ranibizumab for 2 years (which were compared with sham injections in MARINA and with photodynamic therapy in ANCHOR) and not only demonstrated prevention of vision loss in the vast majority of patients, but were the first trials in wet AMD to show a mean improvement in visual acuity (Figure 6-1).[9,10,44-46]

Subsequent studies evaluated the safety and efficacy of ranibizumab with alternative dosing regimens as a way to reduce the frequency and overall number of injections. These regimens included as-needed (pro re nata [PRN]), quarterly dosing, and treat-and-extend strategies.[13,42,47-57] The use of OCT as the basis of PRN dosing was first proposed by the Prospective OCT Imaging of Patients with Neovascular AMD Treated with IntraOcular Ranibizumab (PrONTO) study.[55] This small 2-year trial showed that PRN dosing of intravitreal ranibizumab resulted in visual acuity outcomes comparable with the outcomes from the monthly dosing phase III clinical studies but requiring fewer intravitreal injections during this period.

The HARBOR study was a much larger study (1097 patients with subfoveal wet AMD) that evaluated the efficacy and safety of intravitreal ranibizumab at 0.5 and 2.0 mg administered monthly or PRN following 3 monthly injections. At month 12, mean improvement in visual acuity was similar among all treatment groups, with a mean gain in best corrected visual acuity (BCVA) of 10.1 (0.5 mg monthly), 8.2 (0.5 mg PRN), 9.2 (2.0 mg monthly), and 8.6 (2.0 mg PRN) Early Treatment Diabetic Retinopathy Study (ETDRS) letters, although the PRN dosing group did not meet the set noninferiority endpoint of 4.5 letters. The BCVA gains were achieved with an average of 11.3 (0.5 mg monthly), 7.7 (0.5 mg PRN), 11.2 (2.0 mg monthly), and 6.9 (2.0 mg PRN) injections.[58] Results recently presented for the 2-year HARBOR trial showed maintenance of visual acuity gains in all 4 groups, which suggests that an individualized PRN treatment approach with intravitreal ranibizumab may be used to safely treat patients with wet AMD.[56]

RANIBIZUMAB VERSUS BEVACIZUMAB

Two large randomized clinical trials compared bevacizumab with ranibizumab, as well as monthly vs PRN dosing in patients with wet AMD.[12,13,47,48] The Comparison

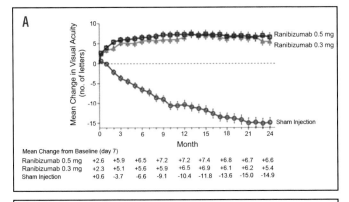

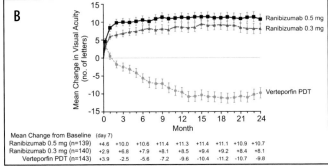

Figure 6-1. (A) Mean change from baseline in visual acuity and Snellen equivalents at 12 and 24 months in the MARINA study. (Reprinted with permission from Rosenfeld PJ, Brown DM, Heier JS, et al. Ranibizumab for neovascular age-related macular degeneration. *N Engl J Med.* 2006;355[14]:1419-1431.) (B) Mean change from baseline in visual acuity at 12 and 24 months in the ANCHOR study. (Reprinted with permission from Brown DM, Michels M, Kaiser PK, et al. Ranibizumab versus verteporfin photodynamic therapy for neovascular age-related macular degeneration: two-year results of the ANCHOR study. *Ophthalmology.* 2009;116[1]:57-65.e5.)

of Age-Related Macular Degeneration Treatment Trial (CATT) was sponsored by the National Eye Institute of the National Institutes of Health. CATT was a prospective, multicenter clinical trial that randomized patients into 4 groups defined by drug (bevacizumab or ranibizumab) and dosing regimen (monthly or PRN). At 1 year, patients assigned to both monthly groups were randomly reassigned to either monthly or PRN treatment (these were called switched regimen groups). Bevacizumab and ranibizumab showed similar effects on visual acuity when administered in the same dosing regimen (bevacizumab was found to be noninferior to ranibizumab after 2 years); however, PRN dosing was not as good as monthly dosing after 2 years (PRN treatment did not meet the noninferiority endpoint compared with monthly dosing) (Figure 6-2A). At 2 years, the mean increase in visual acuity letters from baseline was 8.8 in the ranibizumab-monthly group, 7.8 in the bevacizumab-monthly group, 6.7 in the ranibizumab-PRN group, and 5.0 in the bevacizumab-PRN group (drug $P=.21$; regimen $P=.046$). Mean visual acuity change occurred most in the first year of the study.[12]

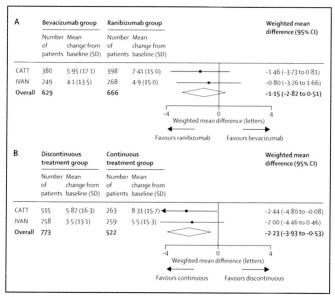

Figure 6-2. Change in best corrected distance visual acuity in the CATT and IVAN trials at 2 years. (A) Change by drug. (B) Change by regimen. 95% confidence intervals represented by bars. (Reprinted with permission from Chakravarthy U, Harding SP, Rogers CA, et al. Alternative treatments to inhibit VEGF in age-related choroidal neovascularisation: 2-year findings of the IVAN randomised controlled trial. *Lancet.* 2013;382[9900]:1258-1267.)

The Inhibition of VEGF in Age-related choroidal Neovascularization (IVAN) trial was a prospective, multicenter, noninferiority clinical trial comparing ranibizumab with bevacizumab for the treatment of treatment-naïve wet AMD and was sponsored by the National Health Service in the United Kingdom. Patients were randomly assigned to intravitreal injections of bevacizumab 1.25 mg or ranibizumab 0.5 mg every month or PRN, with monthly follow-up visits. The 2-year results showed that the drugs had similar efficacy, and when pooled together with the CATT data, there was no significant difference in the 2 drugs. The 2 dosing regimens had similar efficacy as well, although when data from the IVAN and CATT studies were combined, PRN treatment resulted in a statistically significant small loss of efficacy (–2.23 ETDRS letters) compared with monthly treatment (Figure 6-2B).[13]

Two European prospective, multicenter, noninferiority clinical trials also evaluated the safety and efficacy of bevacizumab vs ranibizumab intravitreal injections for the treatment of wet AMD. The GEFAL (Groupe d'Evaluation Français Avastin versus Lucentis) study[59] was performed in 38 French centers and the MANTA (Multicenter Anti-VEGF Trial in Austria) study was performed in 10 Austrian centers.[60,61] In both studies, patients were randomly assigned to one of the 2 drug group and received 3 monthly intravitreal injections followed by monthly visits with PRN treatment for 9 months. Results of the GEFAL and MANTA studies were consistent with other studies, demonstrating that bevacizumab was noninferior to ranibizumab.

Of note, the combined meta-analysis of the IVAN and CATT trials showed a slight difference in the number of nonthromboembolic systemic adverse events (SAEs) between ranibizumab and bevacizumab.[12,13] However, the frequency of adverse events due to thomboembolic events, as well as the overall death rate, was the same between the 2 drugs. The slightly higher rate of SAEs in the bevacizumab group was related mostly to gastrointestinal disorders in the CATT trial, which were not typical of this drug in previously conducted cancer studies using much higher doses of the drug; therefore, it is difficult to make definitive conclusions from this finding. Also of note, in the combined meta-analysis of these 2 trials, the death rate was slightly higher in the noncontinuous group vs the continuous group. It is difficult to interpret this finding because it is not intuitive (ie, less dosing leads to a higher death rate).

AFLIBERCEPT

Aflibercept is a soluble decoy receptor fusion protein consisting of portions of the extracellular domains of human VEGF receptors 1 and 2 fused to the Fc portion of human immunoglobulin G1.[62] Aflibercept binds all isoforms of VEGF-A, VEGF-B, and placental growth factor (PlGF). Pharmacodynamics studies suggest that this molecule should have a longer duration of action in vivo when compared with other available drugs.[11,15,63-72] The use of intravitreal aflibercept in patients with wet AMD was approved by the FDA for patient use in the US in 2011.[73]

Two phase III studies in wet AMD (VEGF Trap-Eye: Investigation of Efficacy and Safety in Wet AMD [VIEW 1 and VIEW 2]) compared monthly and every-2-month dosing of intravitreal aflibercept injection with monthly ranibizumab.[11] In these double-masked, multicenter, noninferiority trials, patients were randomized to intravitreal aflibercept 0.5 mg monthly, 2 mg monthly, 2 mg every 2 months after 3 initial monthly doses, or ranibizumab 0.5 mg given monthly. Results of these studies demonstrated that all aflibercept groups were clinically equivalent (noninferior) to monthly ranibizumab in maintaining visual acuity at week 52. They concluded that aflibercept is an effective treatment for AMD, with the every-2-month regimen offering the potential to reduce the risk from monthly intravitreal injections (Figure 6-3).[11]

During the second year of the study, all patients maintained their drug assignments and were treated using a capped PRN regimen (PRN dosing with a required minimum dosing of every 3 months) in which patients were followed monthly and given a dose of the drug if there was OCT evidence of macular fluid. The visual benefit decreased slightly during the second year of the study. Across treatment groups, mean BCVA gains were 8.3 to 9.3 letters at week 52 and 6.6 to 7.9 letters at week 96. The data showed that all treatment groups with aflibercept and ranibizumab had improved mean overall BCVA through 2 years.[74]

INTRAVITREAL INJECTION PROCEDURE

It is important to minimize both discomfort and the risk of endophthalmitis when performing an intravitreal injection of an anti-VEGF drug. Sterile technique is essential during the procedure, but an operating room is not required. Injections can be conveniently and successfully administered in a normal clinic room without special airflow requirements. Although there is considerable variation in how injections are performed, there are certain steps that are universally accepted as necessary at different stages of the injection procedure.[75]

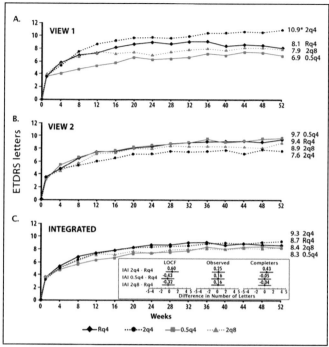

Figure 6-3. Mean change in best corrected visual acuity from baseline to week 52 in (A, B) the individual VIEW studies and (C) the integrated analysis. Values in the line graphs refer to mean changes in the number of letters from baseline at week 52. Only the intravitreal aflibercept 2q4 arm in VIEW 1 was significantly different from ranibizumab (*P=.005 for the difference). The panel inset (integrated analysis) shows the difference in visual acuity between each intravitreal aflibercept arm and ranibizumab (least-square mean with 95% confidence interval) at week 52, using 3 different analyses: by last observation carried forward (LOCF), using observed case data, and by assessing completers. Rq4=0.5 mg ranibizumab monthly; 0.5q4=0.5 mg IAI monthly; 2q4=2 mg IAI monthly; 2q8=2 mg IAI every 2 months after 3 initial monthly doses. Abbreviations: ETDRS, Early Treatment Diabetic Retinopathy Study; IAI, intravitreal aflibercept injection. (Reprinted with permission from Heier JS, Brown DM, Chong V, et al. Intravitreal aflibercept [VEGF trap-eye] in wet age-related macular degeneration. *Ophthalmology.* 2012;119[12]:2537-2548.)

Patient Informed Consent

Patient authorization or agreement is an important step before performing the injection and must be documented in writing. Several minor ocular adverse effects are relatively common after intravitreal injection, including foreign body sensation, subconjunctival hemorrhage, superficial punctate keratopathy, and vitreous floaters.[76,77] Although rare, severe complications such as infectious endophthalmitis, transient noninfectious uveitis, ocular hypertension, retinal tears, rhegmatogenous retinal detachment, and either traumatic or secondary nontraumatic cataract can occur.[76,78] Although major ocular complications of intravitreal injections are infrequent, they can lead to vision loss and blindness; therefore, patients should be counseled appropriately, and an informed consent form should be signed. If using bevacizumab for intraocular use, it is important to remember that the use is off-label, which should be discussed with the patient and included in the informed consent.

Systemic Risk of Anti-Vascular Endothelial Growth Factor Treatment

The systemic risks of intravitreal anti-VEGF medications, if they exist, are small. It is well known that systemic blockade of VEGF with intravenous bevacizumab or aflibercept increases blood pressure and the risk for thromboembolic events, but the amount of anti-VEGF medication that enters the bloodstream after intravitreal injection is minute (systemic anti-VEGF levels, although small, are highest and longest-lasting with bevacizumab and lowest and shortest-lasting with ranibizumab). The CATT and IVAN trials showed no sign that the rate of thromboembolic events was increased by injection of intravitreal anti-VEGF medication, and rates of thromboembolic events with both ranibizumab and bevacizumab were equivalent.[12,13] However, there may be a theoretical slight increase in the risk of thromboembolic events in patients receiving anti-VEGF medications, and, in patients who are at highest risk for these events, it may be worth considering switching to ranibizumab or delaying treatment in the setting of a recent thromboembolic event.

Personal Protective Equipment

The use of gloves during the procedure is common practice, although there is no evidence that gloves reduce the risk of infection. A survey of retina specialists performing intravitreal injection techniques in the United States demonstrated that 58% of them use gloves for this procedure.[79] Of this total, 58% used sterile gloves and 42% used nonsterile new gloves.

The use of a face mask is not established as routine.[80,81] However, in 2011, Wen et al[82] published a study in which a blood agar plate was placed to simulate the position of the patient's eye. The authors showed that wearing a face mask and talking to the patient, turning the head away from the patient and talking, or keeping silent during the injection significantly reduced the rate of bacterial growth when compared with facing the patient and talking without a mask. Oral streptococcal species represented 67% to 83% of bacterial colonies when the authors faced the patient, but only 20% of bacterial colonies when the head was turned.[82] This does not prove that the use of a face mask directly correlates with decreased rates of endophthalmitis, and the use of masks should not be considered standard of care; however, silence during the procedure is recommended.[80,83] In a survey of retina specialists from the United States, most of the participants (59.4%) said that they avoid talking and ask the patient not to speak during the intravitreal injection.[84]

Prophylaxis With Topical Antibiotics

There is no evidence that the use of topical antibiotics reduces the risk of endophthalmitis. Moreover, studies have demonstrated that repeated use of antibiotics for intraocular injections promotes antimicrobial resistance.[85,86]

In an assessment of 3226 ranibizumab injections given between 2 Diabetic Retinopathy Clinical Research (DRCR) Network trials, 3 (0.09%) cases of endophthalmitis were observed, and these eyes had received topical antibiotics for several days after, but not prior to, the injection.[87] With this low reported rate of endophthalmitis, the authors suggest a protocol that uses topical povidone-iodine, a sterile lid speculum, and topical anesthetic without the use of topical antibiotics, sterile gloves, or sterile drape.

An evaluation of 4 DRCR Network trials described 7 cases of endophthalmitis among patients receiving intravitreal injections (ranibizumab or triamcinolone acetonide).[88] Six (0.13%) occurred with the use of topical prophylactic antibiotics among 4694 injections, whereas 1 (0.03%) case occurred without the use of topical antibiotics among 3333 injections. These data confirm the low rate of endophthalmitis in cases of intravitreal injections without the use of prophylactic antibiotics.

Use of Povidone-Iodine

The most common agent used to reduce ocular flora is povidone-iodine, which is safe and inexpensive.[79,89] The application of topical povidone-iodine, a bactericidal agent, is recommended to reduce the risk of endophthalmitis.[90] Povidone-iodine provides microbicidal activity against a broad spectrum of organisms, and anaphylaxis to the compound is exceedingly rare. A wide range of povidone-iodine concentrations (from 0.005% to 10%) have been shown to be bactericidal, and the kill time is as short as 15 to 120 seconds when used at concentrations of 0.1% to 10%.[91] Adverse effects from the use of povidone-iodine on and around the eye include ocular irritation and contact dermatitis.[90,92]

Lid Speculum

Guidelines for intravitreal injection published in 2004 encouraged the use of a speculum to avoid contamination of the needle with the eyelashes or the eyelid margin during the procedure.[93] Excessive manipulation of the lid margin should be avoided to limit expression of bacteria-laden secretions from the meibomian glands and reduce the risk of contamination of the ocular surface.[89]

Anesthesia

There is no evidence for or consensus on the best anesthetic technique to use for intravitreal injection. Four anesthetic techniques are being used among retina specialists at a similar rate: topical anesthetic drops, topical viscous anesthetic drops, topical anesthetic administered on a pledget or cotton tip, and subconjunctival injection of anesthetic.[94]

Yau et al[95] compared 3 topical agents in 93 patients receiving intravitreal ranibizumab for wet AMD. The study was prospective, double-masked, and randomized. Patients received 0.5% tetracaine hydrochloride drops and a 4% lidocaine pledget, 0.5% tetracaine hydrochloride drops alone, or 4% cocaine (+ epinephrine 1/100000) drops alone. The pain experienced by the patient was assessed using a visual analog scale (VAS) immediately postinjection and 15 minutes postinjection. The physician performing the intravitreal injection scored his perception of the patients' pain using the Wong-Baker FACES scale. Results of this study demonstrated no clinical difference in patient pain experience between the 3 topical anesthetic options tested.[95]

During anesthetic preparation, a simple and minimally invasive procedure can lower the intraocular pressure (IOP) spike immediately after the intravitreal injection. The maneuver consists of ocular decompression with a cotton swab, creating a visible indentation in the area of swab application. In a study evaluating the effect of mechanical ocular decompression, the IOP spike was significantly lower ($P < .001$) in the cotton swab compression group (mean IOP, 41.2 mm Hg [range, 21 to 68 mm Hg]) compared with the no-compression group (mean IOP, 46.8 mm Hg [range, 29 to 76 mm Hg]).[96] Mean change in IOP was 25.7 mm Hg (range, 7 to 49 mm Hg) in the compression group and 30.9 mm Hg (range, 13 to 56 mm Hg) in the no-compression group.

Injection Technique

It is recommended to administer anti-VEGF injections through the pars plana, usually in the inferotemporal or superotemporal quadrant, at a distance of 3.5 mm (pseudophakic) or 4 mm (phakic) posterior to the limbus, with the needle directed toward the center of the vitreous cavity. The use of a sterile caliper can help in measuring the correct distance from the limbus. The half-inch needle can be buried to the hub at the time of injection, although the needle is usually inserted one-half to three-quarters of the way into the vitreous cavity. After injection, a sterile cotton swab can be used to cover the site of the injection to avoid drug reflux and vitreous egress.

Postinjection Procedures

Transient increase in IOP is a common and well-described outcome following intravitreal injection of an anti-VEGF drug.[97-103] The acute IOP elevation is related to the volume injected[100,104,105] into the vitreous cavity and can be a risk for short-term occlusion of the central retinal artery.[99] The technique of ocular compression described earlier results in less of an IOP elevation after intravitreal injection and decreases the risk of arterial occlusion.

Optic nerve reperfusion can be assessed and confirmed after intravitreal injection by indirect ophthalmoscopy or testing for the ability to count fingers or hand motion.[93] The routine prophylactic use of an anterior-chamber paracentesis to control postinjection IOP is unnecessary, but the procedure can be considered in cases of prolonged nonperfusion of the optic nerve after intravitreal injection.

Occasionally, over the course of repeated intravitreal anti-VEGF injections, patients may manifest a gradual increase in IOP from baseline. The exact mechanism of action that causes persistent IOP elevation is unknown, but it is most likely related to the pharmacologic properties of the medication,[99,106] which may obstruct outflow[107] or have a toxic effect directly on the trabecular meshwork.[108] The greater number of anti-VEGF injections and shorter interval between the injections are associated with higher IOP, so repeated increases in IOP immediately postinjection may also directly damage the trabecular meshwork.[109,110] Sustained IOP elevation can occur even if the patient has tolerated multiple injections without IOP elevation, and it should be recognized and treated to avoid complications.[107] In patients presenting with ocular hypertension, a glaucoma workup and examination are recommended.[111]

After the intravitreal injection, the patient should receive final instructions, which include all the warning signs of postinjection endophthalmitis. It is extremely important to explain to the patient that he or she needs to contact the ophthalmologist or return for an immediate evaluation in case of worsening eye redness, ocular pain, or decreased vision after the injection.

Injection Regimen

It is known that for virtually all patients with wet AMD, anti-VEGF injections must be given on a regular basis to achieve the best visual outcomes. So far, no treatment regimen has shown better short-term (up to 2 years) visual outcomes than monthly therapy. The PIER study compared monthly injections of ranibizumab to every-3-month dosing of ranibizumab. Despite an initial improvement of visual acuity in both groups, the every-3-month treatment arm underperformed the monthly treatment arm over the course of the trial.[42] However, monthly injections are costly and burdensome to patients, and each injection poses the rare risk of a severe complication; therefore, less frequent injection regimens that can maintain visual improvements are desirable. Data from the CATT and IVAN trials suggest that more frequent dosing of anti-VEGF medication may lead to increased rate of formation of geographic atrophy over time.[12,13] For these reasons, treatment is often individualized for each patient. There are 2 major treatment approaches to accomplish individualized therapy: PRN treatment and treat-and-extend. Another alternative to monthly treatments can be successfully done with aflibercept: 3 monthly injections followed by every-other-month injections.

Monthly injections have been compared with PRN treatment in several randomized clinical trials, and results suggest that PRN treatment results in a sustained visual benefit, although slightly less visual benefit over time compared with monthly treatment.[12,13,56,59-61] It is important to note that the best visual results with PRN treatment are attained when patients are followed monthly in the clinic, with retreatments performed when specific clinical or OCT parameters are noted. Fixed interval therapy with aflibercept every 2 months was compared with fixed interval monthly injections of aflibercept as well as monthly ranibizumab in a randomized trial, and results suggested that the less-frequent dosing of aflibercept was equivalent to both monthly dosing regimens.[11]

Interestingly, in a survey conducted by the American Society of Retina Specialists in 2013, the most common treatment regimen used by retina specialists is treat-and-extend,[84] which has not been evaluated in a prospective, randomized clinical trial. However, studies suggest that visual acuity results are similar to monthly injections.[112,113] In the treat-and-extend regimen, injections are performed monthly until there is no more evidence of fluid on OCT or exudation on biomicroscopic examination or no further improvement in vision or OCT occurs with repeated monthly treatments. The injection interval is then extended by 1 to 2 weeks, the injection is repeated, and, if the OCT and examination continue to show no sign of increased exudation, the next visit is extended by another 1 to 2 weeks. The injection interval can continue to be extended in this fashion as long as there is no sign of exudation on examination or OCT (some investigators suggest not extending the injection interval greater than 3 to 4 months). However, if there appear to be signs of increased exudation on examination or OCT at any visit, the injection interval is shortened by 1 to 2 weeks. If there continue to be signs of exudation, the injection interval is again shortened until there is again no sign of exudation on OCT or examination. Patients may then be maintained on the least-frequent injection regimen necessary to maintain an absence of exudation on OCT or examination.

SUMMARY

Intravitreal injections of anti-VEGF drugs have dramatically improved outcomes for patients with wet AMD. Intravitreal anti-VEGF therapy started with pegaptanib, which was soon replaced by off-label bevacizumab, followed by FDA approval of ranibizumab and, more recently, aflibercept for use in wet AMD. Several clinical trials evaluating the effects of anti-VEGF therapy have been completed, and many others are ongoing. The efficacies of bevacizumab, ranibizumab, and aflibercept appear similar as long as adequate treatment and close follow-up are provided, which may require injections as often as every month. The increasing number of patients undergoing frequent intravitreal injections for wet AMD emphasizes the importance of proper injection technique and follow-up examinations to minimize the risk of endophthalmitis and postinjection IOP elevations.

REFERENCES

1. Ferrara N. Vascular endothelial growth factor: basic science and clinical progress. *Endocr Rev.* 2004;25(4):581-611.

2. Keyt BA, Berleau LT, Nguyen HV, et al. The carboxyl-terminal domain (111-165) of vascular endothelial growth factor is critical for its mitogenic potency. *J Biol Chem.* 1996;271(13):7788-7795.

3. Lee S, Jilani SM, Nikolova GV, Carpizo D, Iruela-Arispe ML. Processing of VEGF-A by matrix metalloproteinases regulates bioavailability and vascular patterning in tumors. *J Cell Biol.* 2005;169(4):681-691.

4. Zhao L, Grob S, Avery R, et al. Common variant in VEGFA and response to anti-VEGF therapy for neovascular age-related macular degeneration. *Curr Mol Med.* 2013;13(6):929-934.

5. Rakic JM, Lambert V, Devy L, et al. Placental growth factor, a member of the VEGF family, contributes to the development of choroidal neovascularization. *Invest Ophthalmol Vis Sci.* 2003;44(7):3186-3193.

6. Adamis AP, Shima DT. The role of vascular endothelial growth factor in ocular health and disease. *Retina.* 2005;25(2):111-118.

7. Huang C, Xu Y, Li X, Wang W. Vascular endothelial growth factor A polymorphisms and age-related macular degeneration: a systematic review and meta-analysis. *Mol Vis.* 2013;19:1211-1221.

8. Cruz-Gonzalez F, Cieza-Borrella C, Cabrillo-Estevez L, Canete-Campos C, Escudero-Dominguez F, Gonzalez-Sarmiento R. VEGF A (rs699947 and rs833061) and VEGFR2 (rs2071559) gene polymorphisms are not associated with AMD susceptibility in a Spanish population. *Curr Eye Res.* 2013;38(12):1274-1277.

9. Rosenfeld PJ, Brown DM, Heier JS, et al. Ranibizumab for neovascular age-related macular degeneration. *N Engl J Med.* 2006;355(14):1419-1431.

10. Brown DM, Michels M, Kaiser PK, Heier JS, Sy JP, Ianchulev T. Ranibizumab versus verteporfin photodynamic therapy for neovascular age-related macular degeneration: two-year results of the ANCHOR study. *Ophthalmology.* 2009;116(1):57-65.e55.

11. Heier JS, Brown DM, Chong V, et al. Intravitreal aflibercept (VEGF trap-eye) in wet age-related macular degeneration. *Ophthalmology.* 2012;119(12):2537-2548.

12. Martin DF, Maguire MG, Fine SL, et al. Ranibizumab and bevacizumab for treatment of neovascular age-related macular degeneration: two-year results. *Ophthalmology.* 2012;119(7):1388-1398.

13. Chakravarthy U, Harding SP, Rogers CA, et al. Alternative treatments to inhibit VEGF in age-related choroidal neovascularisation: 2-year findings of the IVAN randomised controlled trial. *Lancet.* 2013; 283(9900):1258-1267.

14. Rosenfeld PJ. Bevacizumab versus ranibizumab for AMD. *N Engl J Med.* 2011;364(20):1966-1967.

15. Stewart MW. Aflibercept (VEGF-TRAP): the next anti-VEGF drug. *Inflamm Allergy Drug Targets.* 2011;10(6):497-508.

16. American Academy of Ophthalmology Retina Panel. *Preferred Practice Pattern Guidelines: Age-Related Macular Degeneration*. San Francisco, CA: American Academy of Ophthalmology; 2008.

17. D'Amico DJ, Masonson HN, Patel M, et al. Pegaptanib sodium for neovascular age-related macular degeneration: two-year safety results of the two prospective, multicenter, controlled clinical trials. *Ophthalmology*. 2006;113(6):992-1001.e1006.

18. Gragoudas ES, Adamis AP, Cunningham ET Jr, Feinsod M, Guyer DR. Pegaptanib for neovascular age-related macular degeneration. *N Engl J Med*. 2004;351(27):2805-2816.

19. Chakravarthy U, Adamis AP, Cunningham ET Jr, et al. Year 2 efficacy results of 2 randomized controlled clinical trials of pegaptanib for neovascular age-related macular degeneration. *Ophthalmology*. 2006;113(9):1508.e1501-e1525.

20. Doggrell SA. Pegaptanib: the first antiangiogenic agent approved for neovascular macular degeneration. *Expert Opin Pharmacother*. 2005;6(8):1421-1423.

21. Sassa Y, Hata Y. Antiangiogenic drugs in the management of ocular diseases: focus on antivascular endothelial growth factor. *Clin Ophthalmol*. 2010;4:275-283.

22. Yancopoulos GD. Clinical application of therapies targeting VEGF. *Cell*. 2010;143(1):13-16.

23. Hurwitz H, Fehrenbacher L, Novotny W, et al. Bevacizumab plus irinotecan, fluorouracil, and leucovorin for metastatic colorectal cancer. *N Engl J Med*. 2004;350(23):2335-2342.

24. Adding a humanized antibody to vascular endothelial growth factor (Bevacizumab, Avastin) to chemotherapy improves survival in metastatic colorectal cancer. *Clin Colorectal Cancer*. 2003;3(2):85-88.

25. Michels S, Rosenfeld PJ, Puliafito CA, Marcus EN, Venkatraman AS. Systemic bevacizumab (Avastin) therapy for neovascular age-related macular degeneration twelve-week results of an uncontrolled open-label clinical study. *Ophthalmology*. 2005;112(6):1035-1047.

26. Rosenfeld PJ, Moshfeghi AA, Puliafito CA. Optical coherence tomography findings after an intravitreal injection of bevacizumab (avastin) for neovascular age-related macular degeneration. *Ophthalmic Surg Lasers Imaging*. 2005;36(4):331-335.

27. Rich RM, Rosenfeld PJ, Puliafito CA, et al. Short-term safety and efficacy of intravitreal bevacizumab (Avastin) for neovascular age-related macular degeneration. *Retina*. 2006;26(5):495-511.

28. Spaide RF, Laud K, Fine HF, et al. Intravitreal bevacizumab treatment of choroidal neovascularization secondary to age-related macular degeneration. *Retina*. 2006;26(4):383-390.

29. Avery RL, Pieramici DJ, Rabena MD, Castellarin AA, Nasir MA, Giust MJ. Intravitreal bevacizumab (Avastin) for neovascular age-related macular degeneration. *Ophthalmology*. 2006;113(3):363-372.e365.

30. Bashshur ZF, Bazarbachi A, Schakal A, Haddad ZA, El Haibi CP, Noureddin BN. Intravitreal bevacizumab for the management of choroidal neovascularization in age-related macular degeneration. *Am J Ophthalmol*. 2006;142(1):1-9.

31. Geitzenauer W, Michels S, Prager F, et al. Early effects of systemic and intravitreal bevacizumab (avastin) therapy for neovascular age-related macular degeneration [in German]. *Klin Monbl Augenheilkd*. 2006;223(10):822-827.

32. Ladewig MS, Ziemssen F, Jaissle G, et al. Intravitreal bevacizumab for neovascular age-related macular degeneration [in German]. *Ophthalmologe*. 2006;103(6):463-470.

33. Costa RA, Jorge R, Calucci D, Cardillo JA, Melo LA Jr, Scott IU. Intravitreal bevacizumab for choroidal neovascularization caused by AMD (IBeNA Study): results of a phase 1 dose-escalation study. *Invest Ophthalmol Vis Sci*. 2006;47(10):4569-4578.

34. Yoganathan P, Deramo VA, Lai JC, Tibrewala RK, Fastenberg DM. Visual improvement following intravitreal bevacizumab (Avastin) in exudative age-related macular degeneration. *Retina*. 2006;26(9):994-998.

35. Hughes MS, Sang DN. Safety and efficacy of intravitreal bevacizumab followed by pegaptanib maintenance as a treatment regimen for age-related macular degeneration. *Ophthalmic Surg Lasers Imaging*. 2006;37(6):446-454.

36. Aggio FB, Farah ME, Silva WC, Melo GB. Intravitreal bevacizumab for exudative age-related macular degeneration after multiple treatments. *Graefes Arch Clin Exp Ophthalmol*. 2007;245(2):215-220.

37. Chen CY, Wong TY, Heriot WJ. Intravitreal bevacizumab (Avastin) for neovascular age-related macular degeneration: a short-term study. *Am J Ophthalmol.* 2007;143(3):510-512.

38. Giansanti F, Virgili G, Bini A, et al. Intravitreal bevacizumab therapy for choroidal neovascularization secondary to age-related macular degeneration: 6-month results of an open-label uncontrolled clinical study. *Eur J Ophthalmol.* 2007;17(2):230-237.

39. Chen E, Kaiser RS, Vander JF. Intravitreal bevacizumab for refractory pigment epithelial detachment with occult choroidal neovascularization in age-related macular degeneration. *Retina.* 2007;27(4):445-450.

40. Tufail A, Patel PJ, Egan C, et al. Bevacizumab for neovascular age related macular degeneration (ABC Trial): multicentre randomised double masked study. *BMJ.* 2010;340:c2459.

41. Shienbaum G, Flynn HW Jr. Compounding bevacizumab for intravitreal injection: does USP <797> always apply? *Retina.* 2013;33(9):1733-1734.

42. Abraham P, Yue H, Wilson L. Randomized, double-masked, sham-controlled trial of ranibizumab for neovascular age-related macular degeneration: PIER study year 2. *Am J Ophthalmol.* 2010;150(3):315-324.e311.

43. Ferrara N, Damico L, Shams N, Lowman H, Kim R. Development of ranibizumab, an anti-vascular endothelial growth factor antigen binding fragment, as therapy for neovascular age-related macular degeneration. *Retina.* 2006;26(8):859-870.

44. Kaiser PK, Blodi BA, Shapiro H, Acharya NR. Angiographic and optical coherence tomographic results of the MARINA study of ranibizumab in neovascular age-related macular degeneration. *Ophthalmology.* 2007;114(10):1868-1875.

45. Brown DM, Kaiser PK, Michels M, et al. Ranibizumab versus verteporfin for neovascular age-related macular degeneration. *N Engl J Med.* 2006;355(14):1432-1444.

46. Kaiser PK, Brown DM, Zhang K, et al. Ranibizumab for predominantly classic neovascular age-related macular degeneration: subgroup analysis of first-year ANCHOR results. *Am J Ophthalmol.* 2007;144(6):850-857.

47. Martin DF, Maguire MG, Ying GS, Grunwald JE, Fine SL, Jaffe GJ. Ranibizumab and bevacizumab for neovascular age-related macular degeneration. *N Engl J Med.* 2011;364(20):1897-1908.

48. Chakravarthy U, Harding SP, Rogers CA, et al. Ranibizumab versus bevacizumab to treat neovascular age-related macular degeneration: one-year findings from the IVAN randomized trial. *Ophthalmology.* 2012;119(7):1399-1411.

49. Singer MA, Awh CC, Sadda S, et al. HORIZON: an open-label extension trial of ranibizumab for choroidal neovascularization secondary to age-related macular degeneration. *Ophthalmology.* 2012;119(6):1175-1183.

50. Regillo CD, Brown DM, Abraham P, et al. Randomized, double-masked, sham-controlled trial of ranibizumab for neovascular age-related macular degeneration: PIER Study year 1. *Am J Ophthalmol.* 2008;145(2):239-248.

51. Mitchell P, Korobelnik JF, Lanzetta P, et al. Ranibizumab (Lucentis) in neovascular age-related macular degeneration: evidence from clinical trials. *Br J Ophthalmol.* 2010;94(1):2-13.

52. Silva R, Axer-Siegel R, Eldem B, et al. The SECURE study: long-term safety of ranibizumab 0.5 mg in neovascular age-related macular degeneration. *Ophthalmology.* 2013;120(1):130-139.

53. Schmidt-Erfurth U, Eldem B, Guymer R, et al. Efficacy and safety of monthly versus quarterly ranibizumab treatment in neovascular age-related macular degeneration: the EXCITE study. *Ophthalmology.* 2011;118(5):831-839.

54. Holz FG, Amoaku W, Donate J, et al. Safety and efficacy of a flexible dosing regimen of ranibizumab in neovascular age-related macular degeneration: the SUSTAIN study. *Ophthalmology.* 2011;118(4):663-671.

55. Lalwani GA, Rosenfeld PJ, Fung AE, et al. A variable-dosing regimen with intravitreal ranibizumab for neovascular age-related macular degeneration: year 2 of the PrONTO Study. *Am J Ophthalmol.* 2009;148(1):43-58.e41.

56. Busbee B. HARBOR 2-year results support individualized dosing in patients with wet age-related macular degeneration. Paper presented at: American Society of Retina Specialists (ASRS) Meeting; August 2013; Toronto, Canada.

57. Boyer DS, Heier JS, Brown DM, Francom SF, Ianchulev T, Rubio RG. A phase IIIb study to evaluate the safety of ranibizumab in subjects with neovascular age-related macular degeneration. *Ophthalmology.* 2009;116(9):1731-1739.

58. Busbee BG, Ho AC, Brown DM, et al. Twelve-month efficacy and safety of 0.5 mg or 2.0 mg ranibizumab in patients with subfoveal neovascular age-related macular degeneration. *Ophthalmology.* 2013;120(5):1046-1056.

59. Kodjikian L, Souied EH, Mimoun G, et al. Ranibizumab versus bevacizumab for neovascular age-related macular degeneration: results from the GEFAL noninferiority randomized trial. *Ophthalmology.* 2013;120(11):2300-2309.

60. Krebs I, Schmetterer L, Boltz A, et al. A randomised double-masked trial comparing the visual outcome after treatment with ranibizumab or bevacizumab in patients with neovascular age-related macular degeneration. *Br J Ophthalmol.* 2013;97(3):266-271.

61. Ehlers JP. The MANTA 1-year results: the anti-VEGF debate continues. *Br J Ophthalmol.* 2013;97(3):248-250.

62. Holash J, Davis S, Papadopoulos N, et al. VEGF-Trap: a VEGF blocker with potent antitumor effects. *Proceed Natl Acad Sci U S A.* 2002;99(17):11393-11398.

63. Lanzetta P, Mitchell P, Wolf S, Veritti D. Different antivascular endothelial growth factor treatments and regimens and their outcomes in neovascular age-related macular degeneration: a literature review. *Br J Ophthalmol.* 2013;97(12):1497-507.

64. Browning DJ, Kaiser PK, Rosenfeld PJ, Stewart MW. Aflibercept for age-related macular degeneration: a game-changer or quiet addition? *Am J Ophthalmol.* 2012;154(2):222-226.

65. Stewart MW. Clinical and differential utility of VEGF inhibitors in wet age-related macular degeneration: focus on aflibercept. *Clin Ophthalmol.* 2012;6:1175-1186.

66. Stewart MW. Aflibercept (VEGF Trap-eye): the newest anti-VEGF drug. *Br J Ophthalmol.* 2012;96(9):1157-1158.

67. Stewart MW. Aflibercept (VEGF Trap-Eye) for the treatment of exudative age-related macular degeneration. *Expert Rev Clin Pharmacol.* 2013;6(2):103-113.

68. Stewart MW, Grippon S, Kirkpatrick P. Aflibercept. *Nat Rev Drug Discov.* 2012;11(4):269-270.

69. Ohr M, Kaiser PK. Aflibercept in wet age-related macular degeneration: a perspective review. *Ther Adv Chronic Dis.* 2012;3(4):153-161.

70. Semeraro F, Morescalchi F, Duse S, Parmeggiani F, Gambicorti E, Costagliola C. Aflibercept in wet AMD: specific role and optimal use. *Drug Des Devel Ther.* 2013;7:711-722.

71. Nguyen DH, Luo J, Zhang K, Zhang M. Current therapeutic approaches in neovascular age-related macular degeneration. *Disc Med.* 2013;15(85):343-348.

72. Xu D, Kaiser PK. Intravitreal aflibercept for neovascular age-related macular degeneration. *Immunotherapy.* 2013;5(2):121-130.

73. BLA approval. Department of Health and Human Services. http://www.accessdata.fda.gov/drugsatfda_docs/appletter/2011/125387s000ltr.pdf. Published November 18, 2011. Accessed June 17, 2014.

74. Schmidt-Erfurth U, Kaiser PK, Korobelnik JF, et al. Intravitreal aflibercept injection for neovascular age-related macular degeneration: ninety-six-week results of the VIEW studies. *Ophthalmology.* 2014;121(1):193-201.

75. Tailor R, Beasley R, Yang Y, Narendran N. Evaluation of patients' experiences at different stages of the intravitreal injection procedure: what can be improved? *Clin Ophthalmol.* 2011;5:1499-1502.

76. Jager RD, Aiello LP, Patel SC, Cunningham ET Jr. Risks of intravitreous injection: a comprehensive review. *Retina.* 2004;24(5):676-698.

77. Schwartz SG, Flynn HW, Scott IU. Endophthalmitis after intravitreal injections. *Expert Opin Pharmacother.* 2009;10(13):2119-2126.

78. Moshfeghi AA. Endophthalmitis following intravitreal anti-vascular endothelial growth factor injections for neovascular age-related macular degeneration. *Semin Ophthalmol.* 2011;26(3):139-148.

79. Green-Simms AE, Ekdawi NS, Bakri SJ. Survey of intravitreal injection techniques among retinal specialists in the United States. *Am J Ophthalmol.* 2011;151(2):329-332.

80. Schimel AM, Scott IU, Flynn HW Jr. Endophthalmitis after intravitreal injections: should the use of face masks be the standard of care? *Arch Ophthalmol.* 2011;129(12):1607-1609.

81. Shimada H, Hattori T, Mori R, Nakashizuka H, Fujita K, Yuzawa M. Minimizing the endophthalmitis rate following intravitreal injections using 0.25% povidone-iodine irrigation and surgical mask. *Graefes Arch Clin Exp Ophthalmol.* 2013;251(8):1885-1890.

82. Wen JC, McCannel CA, Mochon AB, Garner OB. Bacterial dispersal associated with speech in the setting of intravitreous injections. *Arch Ophthalmol.* 2011;129(12):1551-1554.

83. Stewart MW. Endophthalmitis after injections of anti-vascular endothelial growth factor drugs. *Retina.* 2011;31(10):1981-1982.

84. American Society of Retina Specialists Preferences and Trends Membership Survey, 2013. http://www.asrs.org/asrs-community/pat-survey. Accessed June 17, 2014.

85. Kim SJ, Toma HS. Antimicrobial resistance and ophthalmic antibiotics: 1-year results of a longitudinal controlled study of patients undergoing intravitreal injections. *Arch Ophthalmol.* 2011;129(9):1180-1188.

86. Yin VT, Weisbrod DJ, Eng KT, et al. Antibiotic resistance of ocular surface flora with repeated use of a topical antibiotic after intravitreal injection. *JAMA Ophthalmol.* 2013;131(4):456-461.

87. Bhavsar AR, Googe JM Jr, Stockdale CR, et al. Risk of endophthalmitis after intravitreal drug injection when topical antibiotics are not required: the diabetic retinopathy clinical research network laser-ranibizumab-triamcinolone clinical trials. *Arch Ophthalmol.* 2009;127(12):1581-1583.

88. Bhavsar AR, Stockdale CR, Ferris FL III, Brucker AJ, Bressler NM, Glassman AR. Update on risk of endophthalmitis after intravitreal drug injections and potential impact of elimination of topical antibiotics. *Arch Ophthalmol.* 2012;130(6):809-810.

89. Kim SJ, Chomsky AS, Sternberg P Jr. Reducing the risk of endophthalmitis after intravitreous injection. *JAMA Ophthalmol.* 2013;131(5):674-675.

90. Speaker MG, Menikoff JA. Prophylaxis of endophthalmitis with topical povidone-iodine. *Ophthalmology.* 1991;98(12):1769-1775.

91. Wykoff CC, Flynn HW Jr, Rosenfeld PJ. Prophylaxis for endophthalmitis following intravitreal injection: antisepsis and antibiotics. *Am J Ophthalmol.* 2011;152(5):717-719.e712.

92. Wykoff CC, Flynn HW Jr, Han DP. Allergy to povidone-iodine and cephalosporins: the clinical dilemma in ophthalmic use. *Am J Ophthalmol.* 2011;151(1):4-6.

93. Aiello LP, Brucker AJ, Chang S, et al. Evolving guidelines for intravitreous injections. *Retina.* 2004;24(5 Suppl):S3-S19.

94. Prenner JL. Anesthesia for intravitreal injection. *Retina.* 2011;31(3):433-434.

95. Yau GL, Jackman CS, Hooper PL, Sheidow TG. Intravitreal injection anesthesia: comparison of different topical agents: a prospective randomized controlled trial. *Am J Ophthalmol.* 2011;151(2):333-337.e332.

96. Gregori NZ, Weiss MJ, Goldhardt R, et al. Ocular decompression with cotton swabs lowers intraocular pressure elevation after intravitreal injection [published online ahead of print April 29, 2013]. *J Glaucoma.*

97. Aref AA. Management of immediate and sustained intraocular pressure rise associated with intravitreal antivascular endothelial growth factor injection therapy. *Curr Opin Ophthalmol.* 2012;23(2):105-110.

98. Hollands H, Wong J, Bruen R, Campbell RJ, Sharma S, Gale J. Short-term intraocular pressure changes after intravitreal injection of bevacizumab. *Can J Ophthalmol.* 2007;42(6):807-811.

99. Falkenstein IA, Cheng L, Freeman WR. Changes of intraocular pressure after intravitreal injection of bevacizumab (avastin). *Retina.* 2007;27(8):1044-1047.

100. Bakri SJ, Pulido JS, McCannel CA, Hodge DO, Diehl N, Hillemeier J. Immediate intraocular pressure changes following intravitreal injections of triamcinolone, pegaptanib, and bevacizumab. *Eye (Lond).* 2009;23(1):181-185.

101. Hariprasad SM, Shah GK, Blinder KJ. Short-term intraocular pressure trends following intravitreal pegaptanib (Macugen) injection. *Am J Ophthalmol.* 2006;141(1):200-201.

102. Gismondi M, Salati C, Salvetat ML, Zeppieri M, Brusini P. Short-term effect of intravitreal injection of Ranibizumab (Lucentis) on intraocular pressure. *J Glaucoma.* 2009;18(9):658-661.

103. Kim JE, Mantravadi AV, Hur EY, Covert DJ. Short-term intraocular pressure changes immediately after intravitreal injections of anti-vascular endothelial growth factor agents. *Am J Ophthalmol.* 2008;146(6):930-934.e931.

104. Frenkel RE, Mani L, Toler AR, Frenkel MP. Intraocular pressure effects of pegaptanib (Macugen) injections in patients with and without glaucoma. *Am J Ophthalmol.* 2007;143(6):1034-1035.

105. Frenkel MP, Haji SA, Frenkel RE. Effect of prophylactic intraocular pressure-lowering medication on intraocular pressure spikes after intravitreal injections. *Arch Ophthalmol.* 2010;128(12):1523-1527.

106. Segal O, Ferencz JR, Cohen P, Nemet AY, Nesher R. Persistent elevation of intraocular pressure following intravitreal injection of bevacizumab. *Isr Med Assoc J.* 2013;15(7):352-355.

107. Tseng JJ, Vance SK, Della Torre KE, et al. Sustained increased intraocular pressure related to intravitreal antivascular endothelial growth factor therapy for neovascular age-related macular degeneration. *J Glaucoma.* 2012;21(4):241-247.

108. Martel JN, Han Y, Lin SC. Severe intraocular pressure fluctuation after intravitreal anti-vascular endothelial growth factor injection. *Ophthalmic Surg Lasers Imaging.* 2011;42 Online:e100-e102.

109. Hoang QV, Mendonca LS, Della Torre KE, Jung JJ, Tsuang AJ, Freund KB. Effect on intraocular pressure in patients receiving unilateral intravitreal anti-vascular endothelial growth factor injections. *Ophthalmology.* 2012;119(2):321-326.

110. Mathalone N, Arodi-Golan A, Sar S, et al. Sustained elevation of intraocular pressure after intravitreal injections of bevacizumab in eyes with neovascular age-related macular degeneration. *Graefes Arch Clin Exp Ophthalmol.* 2012;250(10):1435-1440.

111. Abedi G, Adelman RA, Salim S. Incidence and management of elevated intraocular pressure with antivascular endothelial growth factor agents. *Semin Ophthalmol.* 2013;28(3):126-130.

112. Shienbaum G, Gupta OP, Fecarotta C, Patel AH, Kaiser RS, Regillo CD. Bevacizumab for neovascular age-related macular degeneration using a treat-and-extend regimen: clinical and economic impact. *Am J Ophthalmol.* 2012;153(3):468-473.

113. Gupta OP, Shienbaum G, Patel AH, Fecarotta C, Kaiser RS, Regillo CD. A treat and extend regimen using ranibizumab for neovascular age-related macular degeneration clinical and economic impact. *Ophthalmology.* 2010;117(11):2134-2140.

7

THERMAL LASER AND PHOTODYNAMIC THERAPY

Llewelyn J. Rao, MD and Lawrence J. Singerman, MD, FACS

Currently, there is no cure for age-related macular degeneration (AMD). The visual devastation from the neovascular (wet) form of this disease has inspired a tremendous amount of research into pharmacologic and surgical therapies. Intravitreal anti-vascular endothelial growth factor (anti-VEGF) injection regimens have drastically changed the treatment algorithm of the vitreoretinal specialist over the past 10 years. Although this treatment modality has become the standard of care for wet AMD, there is still a role for thermal laser and photodynamic therapy (PDT) in select patients. This chapter will focus on these 2 laser therapies for wet AMD.

Thermal laser treatment for choroidal neovascularization (CNV) involves targeted photocoagulation and tissue destruction of CNV membranes. The immediate disadvantage of this treatment is the creation of an absolute scotoma in the treated area. The long-term disadvantage of thermal laser treatment is a high recurrence rate of CNV; therefore, its use is now limited to select cases of extrafoveal CNV, and it is typically used in conjunction with anti-VEGF therapy.

PDT involves the intravenous infusion of a photosensitizing drug, such as verteporfin (Visudyne; Novartis AG), followed by the laser-activated destruction of targeted tissue. The therapeutic effects occur as the laser, whose wavelength corresponds to the absorption peak of the drug, activates and excites the photosensitizer molecules. Unlike thermal laser photocoagulation, PDT does not produce heat damage; therefore, it is sometimes referred to as cold laser. The excited molecules transfer their energy to surrounding tissue via the free radical mechanism, forming cytotoxic intermediates that rapidly oxidize surrounding cellular structures. Thromboxane, histamines, and tumor necrosis factors mediate tissue damage, whereas platelet aggregation, vasoconstriction, and immunologic effects induce direct endothelial damage. Through this mechanism, vessels undergo thrombosis.[1,2]

PDT treatment is selective in 2 ways. First, the intravascular medication is more likely to affect rapidly dividing cells, such as that which occurs with CNV. Second, the medication is activated only within the laser-targeted area. The vascular closure does not occur immediately. The permeability of the CNV can actually increase in the initial 24 hours,

Duker JS, Witkin AJ, eds.
Age-Related Macular Degeneration:
Current Management (pp. 111-119)
© 2015 Taylor & Francis Group

whereas occlusion typically follows over the first week. Retreatment with PDT at more-than-3-month intervals is possible and has been evaluated in the clinical trials discussed in this chapter.

THERMAL LASER

Summary of Prior Trials and Treatment Techniques

The Macular Photocoagulation Studies (MPS) were the landmark randomized, controlled clinical trials that evaluated thermal laser treatment of CNV.[3-13] In these trials, fluorescein angiography (FA) was obtained to identify well-demarcated CNV. Severe visual loss was defined as a loss of 6 or more lines of best corrected visual acuity (BCVA). Some key points from the MPS studies are summarized in this section.

The Argon Macular Photocoagulation Study (1979 to 1988) evaluated the treatment of extrafoveal (200 to 2500 μm from the center of the foveal avascular zone [FAZ]) CNV.[3-5] Argon laser was applied over the CNV, extending 100 to 125 μm beyond its borders. If the lesion extended within 200 to 300 μm of the center of the FAZ, treatment beyond the lesion was not required. The laser spot size was 200 to 500 μm, with a duration of 0.5 seconds. If the treatment was within 350 μm of the FAZ, the burns were decreased to 100 μm in size, and the duration was decreased to 0.1 to 0.2 seconds. Peripapillary CNV was included if the treated area would spare at least 1.5 clock-hours of the peripapillary nerve fiber layer. Severe visual loss occurred in 25% of treated patients at 6 months, 52% at 3 years, and 46% at 5 years. Untreated patients in the study had severe visual loss at rates of 60%, 68%, and 64%, respectively. CNV recurred in 54% of treated patients by 5 years.[3-5]

The Krypton Macular Photocoagulation Study (1982 to 1991) was implemented to assess the treatment of juxtafoveal (1 to 199 μm from the center of the FAZ) CNV or CNV greater than 200 μm from the FAZ, with adjacent blood or pigment extending within 200 μm of the FAZ.[6-8] Krypton red laser was applied and extended for 100 μm beyond the lesion margin, except on the foveal side of the lesion. After 3-year follow-up, severe visual loss had occurred in 49% of treated patients, compared with 58% of untreated patients. Persistent CNV occurred in 32% of patients, whereas recurrent CNV occurred in 41.7% of patients by 5 years.[6-8]

The Foveal Photocoagulation Study (1986 to 1994) evaluated focal laser treatment in patients with subfoveal CNV.[9-11] Eligibility criteria included CNV less than 3.5 MPS disc areas, with most of the lesion composed of classic or occult CNV. Patients were randomized to either krypton red or argon green laser. Treatment was applied 100 μm beyond the lesion margin. Severe visual loss at 3 months occurred more frequently with treatment compared with observation (20% vs 11%, respectively). However, an eventual benefit in treated eyes over the long term was noted compared with observation. At 24 months, severe visual loss occurred in 20% of treated eyes compared with 37% of untreated eyes. This difference was even greater at 4 years, with 22% of treated eyes and 47% of untreated eyes experiencing severe visual loss. The recurrence rate in the treated group was 51%, and most of these recurrent lesions involved the subfoveal region.[9-11]

How Thermal Laser Is Used in the Anti-Vascular Endothelial Growth Factor Era

The use of thermal laser for CNV has dramatically decreased with the advent of intravitreal anti-VEGF injections. The retinal physician no longer has to engage in the difficult discussion of how thermal laser treatment to subfoveal CNV will cause a decline in vision initially, with less visual loss in the long term than the natural history of the disease.

Thermal laser is rarely used as a primary treatment for juxtafoveal or subfoveal CNV; it is now primarily used for the treatment of extrafoveal lesions, with the peripapillary region being one of the more common locations. These lesions must be well defined with fluorescein and/or indocyanine green angiography. If adequately treated, extrafoveal CNVs may remain controlled for extended periods of time, without the need for monthly intravitreal injections (Figure 7-1). After thermal laser, a high rate of recurrence exists[5]; therefore, it is most useful in combination with anti-VEGF therapy as a way to decrease the need for intravitreal injections and limit the incidence of possible complications from frequent injections.

The 2013 Preferences and Trends (PAT) Survey of the American Society of Retinal Specialists (ASRS) asked responders how they would manage a one-half-disc-area, extrafoveal, well-defined CNV secondary to AMD, with visual acuity of 20/25.[12] US responders preferred anti-VEGF injections alone (52.1%); combination therapy of anti-VEGF injections followed by possible laser photocoagulation if the lesion size decreased (30.4%); laser photocoagulation alone (12.4%); and laser photocoagulation followed by anti-VEGF injections (3.1%).

PHOTODYNAMIC THERAPY

Summary of Prior Trials

Two multicenter, randomized, and double-masked clinical trials—the Treatment of AMD With Photodynamic Therapy (TAP) study[13-15] and the Verteporfin in Photodynamic Therapy (VIP) study[16]—evaluated the effectiveness of PDT with verteporfin. Both studies excluded eyes with previous subfoveal laser photocoagulation and those with a lesion diameter larger than 5400 μm.

The TAP study examined subfoveal CNV secondary to AMD in which the CNV was 50% or more of the lesion; the CNV had to have a classic component.[13-15] PDT was allowed every 3 months for 2 years in the presence of persistent leakage or recurrence on FA. After 12-month follow-up, 61.2% of verteporfin-treated eyes, compared with 46.4% of eyes given a placebo, lost less than 15 letters ($P<.001$). Eyes treated with verteporfin were more likely than eyes treated with placebo to have an improvement of one or more lines of vision (16% vs 7%). The average change in BCVA showed verteporfin to be superior to placebo by 1.3 lines at 12 months.

In eyes with 100% classic CNV, 23% of those treated with verteporfin, compared with 73% of those given a placebo, lost 3 or more lines of visual acuity ($P<.001$). In predominantly classic CNV (classic component 50% or more of the lesion), 33% of eyes receiving verteporfin lost 3 or more lines at 12

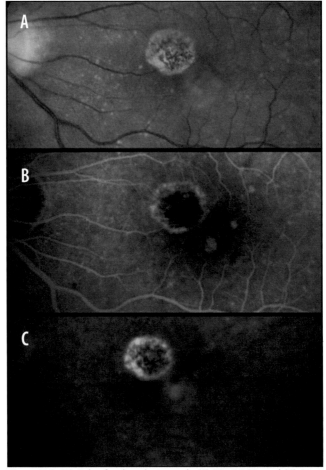

Figure 7-1. (A) Color fundus photograph, (B) FA at 0:28, and (C) FA at 6:20 show scarring superonasally to the fovea secondary to thermal laser treatment for CNV conducted 1 year prior. New CNV lesion is seen inferotemporally to the fovea. Visual acuity before and after the thermal laser treatment was stable at 20/20.

months, compared with 61% of the placebo group. No appreciable visual benefit was seen in eyes with minimally classic CNV (classic component less than 50% of lesion).

Two-year results of the TAP study showed that 53% of the treated eyes lost less than 3 lines of vision, compared with 38% from the placebo group. For predominantly classic lesions at baseline, 59% of the treated eyes lost less than 3 lines of vision, compared with 31% from the placebo group. For minimally classic lesions, no statistically significant difference was noted between the treatment (47.5%) and placebo (44.2%) groups. The mean number of PDT treatments was 3.5 in the first year and 2.3 in the second year.[13,14] When the TAP study was extended into an open-label study for another 3 years, no additional safety concerns with multiple PDT treatments were identified.[15]

The VIP study enrolled patients with CNV secondary to pathologic myopia and occult subfoveal CNV secondary to AMD.[16] Eligibility criteria included disease progression with subretinal hemorrhage, vision loss, or increase in CNV size during a 12-week screening period. Patients with classic CNV were included if they had an Early Treatment Diabetic Retinopathy Study visual acuity score of at least 70 letters (Snellen equivalent 20/40).

At 1 year, no significant difference was noted in vision loss of less than 15 letters between the verteporfin group and the placebo group. At 2 years, 46% of the verteporfin group lost less than 15 letters, compared with 33% from the placebo group. Patients with occult CNV experienced a benefit with verteporfin treatment when the lesion was either less than 4 MPS disc diameters or when the visual acuity was 20/50 or worse. The mean number of PDT treatments was 3.1 in the first year and 1.9 in the second year.[16]

Treatment Technique and Side Effects

Verteporfin is currently the only photosensitizer drug approved by the US Food and Drug Administration for ocular PDT. Verteporfin comes in a powder, which must be reconstituted with 7 mL of sterile water to provide a 7.5 mL solution containing 2 mg/mL verteporfin for injection. The volume of reconstituted verteporfin required to achieve the desired dose of 6 mg/m^2 per body surface area is calculated with a chart provided with the medication, and this amount is withdrawn from the vial and diluted with 5% dextrose, for a total infusion volume of 30 mL. The 30 mL infusion volume is then administered intravenously over 10 minutes at a rate of 3 mL per minute.[17]

The greatest linear dimension (GLD) of the lesion is calculated by FA and color fundus photography. Treatment spot size should be 1000 μm larger than the GLD of the lesion. The maximum spot size used in clinical trials was 6400 μm. At least 200 μm should be between the optic disc and the treatment spot. The nonthermal diode laser (689 nm) is administered for 83 seconds, beginning 15 minutes after the start of the 10-minute intravenous infusion. Standard PDT consists of 50 J/cm^2 dosage and 600 mW/cm^2 intensity.[17]

When PDT was first used, acute severe vision loss sometimes occurred with full fluence, usually due to choroidal hypoperfusion. To limit the toxicity of PDT, fluence may be reduced by either decreasing the power of laser light (less than 50 J/cm^2) or reducing the overall treatment time (less than 83 seconds). Studies have demonstrated that reduced-fluence PDT has similar therapeutic efficacy for CNV but potentially decreases the amount of choroidal toxicity seen with standard-fluence PDT. Many practitioners now use reduced fluence (typically half fluence) to avoid this complication.

Temporary photosensitivity may be present for 5 days after treatment; therefore, patients are instructed to avoid sunlight for that amount of time and to wear sunglasses when outdoors. Other side effects can include pain, swelling, bleeding, or inflammation at the site where the verteporfin medicine is injected. Some people also experience temporary low back pain at the time of intravenous infusion of the medicine.

How Photodynamic Therapy Is Used in the Anti-Vascular Endothelial Growth Factor Era

According to the package insert, verteporfin for injection in PDT is indicated for predominantly classic subfoveal CNV due to AMD, pathologic myopia, or presumed ocular histoplasmosis.[17] As with thermal laser, the use of PDT has greatly decreased since anti-VEGF injections have become the mainstay of treatment for wet AMD. In select

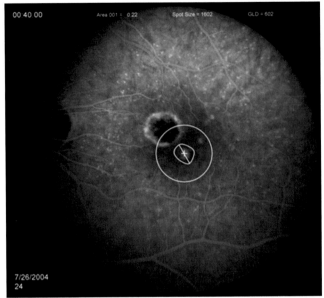

Figure 7-2. FA with spot size and GLD calculation noted at the top. The CNV is outlined in the inner white circle. The outer white circle marks the treatment area, which is extended 1000 μm beyond the GLD of the lesion. Visual acuity remained at 20/20 before and after PDT treatment.

patients, PDT may stop CNV activity for an extended length of time (Figures 7-2 to 7-4). Combination therapy involving PDT, anti-VEGF, and/or intravitreal steroid injection has been studied, but it remains incompletely evaluated.[18-23] Combination therapy with PDT and anti-VEGF therapy to decrease the total number of intravitreal injections has been investigated, but generally no visual benefit has been found compared with anti-VEGF monotherapy.[24,25] Combination therapy with PDT may be most beneficial in patients who are inadequately responsive to anti-VEGF treatment (discussed in more detail in Chapter 9).

The 2013 ASRS PAT survey asked responders what percentage of their patients with wet AMD had been given PDT over the past year.[12] US responders stated that 53.9% had not used it and 44.5% had used it in 1% to 20% of their patients. In addition, the PAT survey asked about management choices for a 1-disc area of subfoveal CNV due to wet AMD, with visual acuity of 20/100. Only 0.4% of US responders listed PDT plus anti-VEGF injection, and only another 0.4% listed those plus steroids.

SUMMARY

Thermal laser therapy and photodynamic therapy have been proven to halt disease progression in many patients with wet AMD. Recurrence of disease activity is well documented in spite of these treatments. Anti-VEGF therapy has now become the standard of care for wet AMD, but combination treatment, consisting of laser (thermal laser or PDT) and anti-VEGF injection therapy, may be useful in certain patients to

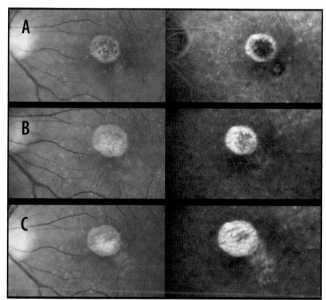

Figure 7-3. Color fundus photographs (left) and FAs (right) at (A) 2 months, (B) 1 year, and (C) 3 years after PDT treatment in the same patient shown in Figures 7-1 and 7-2.

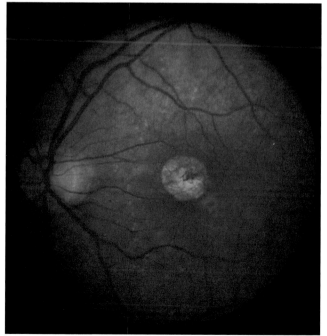

Figure 7-4. Color fundus photograph of the same patient 10 years after thermal laser and 9 years after PDT demonstrates stability in the area of thermal laser, as well as PDT treatment. Visual acuity remained stable at 20/20.

reduce the number of injections required to suppress disease activity or in patients who do not adequately respond to anti-VEGF therapy alone.

REFERENCES

1. Schmidt-Erfurth U, Hasan T, Gargoudas E, Michaud N, Flotte TJ, Birngruber R. Vascular targeting in photodynamic occlusion of subretinal vessels. *Ophthalmologica*. 1994;101:1953-1961.

2. Schmidt-Erfurth U, Laqua H, Schlotzer-Schrehard U, Viestenz A, Naumann GO. Histopathological changes following photodynamic therapy in human eyes. *Arch Ophthalmol*. 2002;120:835-844.

3. Macular Photocoagulation Study Group. Argon laser photocoagulation for senile macular degeneration: results of a randomized clinical trial. *Arch Ophthalmol*. 1982;100:912-918.

4. Macular Photocoagulation Study Group. Argon laser photocoagulation for neovascular maculopathy: three-year results from randomized clinical trials. *Arch Ophthalmol*. 1986;104:694-701.

5. Macular Photocoagulation Study Group. Argon laser photocoagulation for neovascular maculopathy: five-year results from randomized clinical trials. *Arch Ophthalmol*. 1991;109:1109-1114.

6. Macular Photocoagulation Study Group. Krypton laser photocoagulation for neovascular lesions of age-related macular degeneration: results of a randomized clinical trial. *Arch Ophthalmol*. 1990;108:816-824.

7. Macular Photocoagulation Study Group. Persistent and recurrent neovascularization after krypton laser photocoagulation for neovascular lesions of age-related macular degeneration. *Arch Ophthalmol*. 1990;108:825-831.

8. Macular Photocoagulation Study Group. Laser photocoagulation for juxtafoveal choroidal neovascularization: five-year results from randomized clinical trials. *Arch Ophthalmol*. 1994;112:500-509.

9. Macular Photocoagulation Study Group. Laser photocoagulation of subfoveal neovascular lesions in age-related macular degeneration: results of a randomized clinical trial. *Arch Ophthalmol*. 1991;109:1220-1231.

10. Macular Photocoagulation Study Group. Laser photocoagulation of subfoveal neovascular lesions of age-related macular degeneration: updated findings from two clinical trials. *Arch Ophthalmol*. 1993;111:1200-1209.

11. Macular Photocoagulation Study Group. Laser photocoagulation of subfoveal neovascular lesions of age-related macular degeneration: guidelines for evaluation and treatment in the Macular Photocoagulation Study. *Arch Ophthalmol*. 1991;109:1242-1257.

12. Stone TW, Mittra RA, eds. *ASRS 2013 Preferences and Trends Survey*. Chicago, IL; ASRS:2013.

13. Treatment of Age-Related Macular Degeneration With Photodynamic Therapy (TAP) Study Group. Photodynamic therapy of subfoveal choroidal neovascularization in age-related macular degeneration with verteporfin: one-year results of 2 randomized clinical trials—TAP report [published correction appears in *Arch Ophthalmol*. 2000;118:488]. *Arch Ophthalmol*. 1999;117:1329-1345.

14. Treatment of Age-Related Macular Degeneration With Photodynamic Therapy (TAP) Study Group. Photodynamic therapy of subfoveal choroidal neovascularization in age-related macular degeneration with verteporfin: two-year results of 2 randomized clinical trials—TAP report 2. *Arch Ophthalmol*. 2001;119:198-207.

15. Treatment of Age-Related Macular Degeneration With Photodynamic Therapy (TAP) Study Group. Verteporfin therapy for subfoveal choroidal neovascularization in age-related macular degeneration: three-year results of an open-label extension of 2 randomized clinical trials—TAP report no. 5. *Arch Ophthalmol*. 2002;120:1307-1314.

16. Verteporfin in Photodynamic Therapy (VIP) Study Group. Verteporfin therapy of subfoveal choroidal neovascularization in age-related macular degeneration: 2-year results of a randomized clinical trial including lesions with occult with no classic choroidal neovascularization—VIP report 2. *Am J Ophthalmol*. 2001;131:541-560.

17. Visudyne (verteporfin for injection) [package insert]. Bridgewater, NJ: Valeant Pharmaceuticals; 2010.

18. Antoszyk AN, Tuomi L, Chung CY, Singh A; FOCUS Study Group. Ranibizumab combined with verteporfin photodynamic therapy in neovascular age-related macular degeneration (FOCUS): year 2 results. *Am J Ophthalmol.* 2008;145:862-874.

19. Augustin A. Triple therapy for choroidal neovascularization due to age related macular degeneration: verteporfin PDT, bevacizumab, and dexamethasone. *Retina.* 2007;27:133-140.

20. Bakri SJ, Couch SM, McCannel CA, Edwards AO. Same-day triple therapy with photodynamic therapy, intravitreal dexamethasone, and bevacizumab in wet age-related macular degeneration. *Retina.* 2009;29:573-578.

21. Bashshur ZF, Schakal AR, El-Mollayess GM, Arafat S, Jaafar D, Salti HI. Ranibizumab monotherapy versus single-session verteporfin photodynamic therapy combined with as-needed ranibizumab treatment for the management of neovascular age-related macular degeneration. *Retina.* 2011;31:636-644.

22. Lazic R, Gabric N. Verteporfin therapy and intravitreal bevacizumab combined and alone in choroidal neovascularization due to age-related macular degeneration. *Ophthalmology.* 2007;114;1179-1185.

23. Potter MJ, Claudio CC, Szabo SM. A randomized trial of bevacizumab and reduced light dose photodynamic therapy in age-related macular degeneration: the VIA study. *Br J Ophthalmol.* 2010;94:174-179.

24. Kaiser PK, Boyer DS, Cruess AF, Slakter JS, Pilz S, Weisberger A; DENALI Study Group. Verteporfin plus ranibizumab for choroidal neovascularization in age-related macula degeneration: twelve month results of the DENALI study. *Ophthalmology,* 2012;119:1001-1010.

25. Larsen M, Schmidt-Erfurth U, Lanzetta P, et al; MONT BLANC Study Group. Verteporfin plus ranibizumab for choroidal neovascularization in age-related macula degeneration: twelve-month MONT BLANC study results. *Ophthalmology.* 2012;110;992-1000.

8

Treatment Failures

Nonresponders, Tolerance, and Tachyphylaxis

Christopher J. Brady, MD and Chirag P. Shah, MD, MPH

With US Food and Drug Administration approval of intravitreal ranibizumab and aflibercept and the widespread off-label usage of bevacizumab for the management of neovascular (wet) age-related macular degeneration (AMD), retina physicians and their patients entered into a new era in the management of the most common cause of vision loss in the developed world. Despite the remarkable success of these therapies in pivotal clinical trials and in clinical practice, there are individuals who do not achieve the same improvement in vision. For example, in both the Minimally Classic/Occult Trial of the Anti-VEGF Antibody Ranibizumab in the Treatment of Neovascular AMD (MARINA)[1] and Anti-VEGF Antibody for the Treatment of Predominantly Classic Choroidal Neovascularization in AMD (ANCHOR)[2] phase III clinical trials for ranibizumab, 10% of participants who received the 0.5-mg dose lost 15 or more letters of best corrected visual acuity at 2 years. In addition, although 33.3% and 41% of participants improved by 15 or more letters after 2 years in the MARINA and ANCHOR trials, respectively, 22.3% had no improvement in the MARINA study (the value was not reported in the ANCHOR study). Likewise, in the VEGF Trap-Eye: Investigation of Efficacy and Safety in Wet AMD 1 and 2 (VIEW-1/VIEW-2) 12-month report on the phase III trial of aflibercept for AMD, approximately 5% of patients treated with either aflibercept or ranibizumab lost 15 or more letters of visual acuity.[3] Although a strict definition of persistent fluid was used in the Comparison of Age-Related Treatments Trial (CATT), 53.2% and 70.9% of participants demonstrated persistent fluid after 1 year of ranibizumab and bevacizumab, respectively,[4] indicating that a large number of patients continue to have residual disease activity despite frequent treatment.

Importantly, the proportion of participants who lost 15 or more letters in the pivotal trials for ranibizumab doubled between the first and second year of follow-up,[1,2] indicating that there may be an additional subset of patients who are not able to maintain high levels of improvement or stabilization over longer periods of time with continued monthly intravitreal anti-vascular endothelial growth factor (anti-VEGF) injections. When faced with a patient who does not exhibit the expected response to a standard regimen, clinicians do not have the same high level of evidence-based directives to guide

Duker JS, Witkin AJ, eds.
Age-Related Macular Degeneration:
Current Management (pp. 121-128)
© 2015 Taylor & Francis Group

their decision making when contrasted to the information available to guide initial therapy. Ultimately, the clinician must use his or her judgment to choose between 3 practical options, which are usually applied in the following order:

- Switch the anti-VEGF agent
- Increase the dosage or frequency of therapy
- Combine anti-VEGF injection with another modality, such as photodynamic therapy

SWITCHING ANTI-VASCULAR ENDOTHELIAL GROWTH FACTOR AGENTS

Several reports suggest a reduced response to anti-VEGF therapy over time,[5] which may be a manifestation of *tolerance* if the loss of response is gradual but responsive to increasing dosing or dosing frequency or *tachyphylaxis* if the loss of response is rapid and reverses after a decrease in dosing interval. Both tolerant and tachyphylactic eyes may respond to switching to an alternative anti-VEGF agent. In one report, 26 eyes in 25 patients treated initially with either bevacizumab (10 eyes) or ranibizumab (16 eyes) were then switched to the other agent.[6] After a mean of 2.75 injections, 81% of eyes had an anatomic response to the new agent. Visual acuity outcomes were reported but not formally analyzed, although some of the patients who were reported to have an anatomic response to the switch actually had a decrease in visual acuity.[6]

Because aflibercept is the most recently approved anti-VEGF agent for the treatment of wet AMD, a number of retrospective reports on switching patients who had failed either ranibizumab or bevacizumab therapy have recently become available.[7-12] Each report defined the treatment failure slightly differently, but the common theme was that after switching, many patients experienced an anatomical improvement, if not always a visual acuity gain (Figures 8-1 to 8-6). In a review of 36 eyes in 31 patients at the University of Iowa, 50% of eyes showed a reduction in either subretinal or intraretinal fluid, with a mean decrease in central macular thickness (CMT) of 65 μm after 3 injections.[7] In this population, there was no significant change in visual acuity.[7] A cohort of 96 eyes in 85 patients who were switched to aflibercept because of inadequate disease control or intolerance to prior anti-VEGF therapy were analyzed after 4 aflibercept injections.[8] In this group, 49% showed improvement in macular edema on optical coherence tomography (OCT), but there was similarly no significant gain in visual acuity.[8]

Another cohort of 102 eyes in 94 patients received a mean of 3.8 aflibercept injections after receiving a mean of 20.4 injections of either bevacizumab or ranibizumab.[9] In this group, 39% of eyes showed an improvement or resolution of intraretinal and subretinal fluid, although there was no significant gain in visual acuity. Interestingly, the injection interval was extended to 7.3 weeks compared with 5.9 weeks prior to starting aflibercept. In addition, the investigators compared results among refractory and recurrent subgroups. The refractory patients seemed to have a greater reduction in CMT but less tolerance to extension, whereas the recurrent patients had less improvement in CMT but were able to be extended from 7.21 weeks to 9.47 weeks. Given the retrospective nature of this report, it is hard to know whether strict monthly aflibercept therapy would have significantly affected the results.[9]

Another group reviewed the records of 28 eyes in 28 patients who were switched to aflibercept due to persistent fluid after an average of 20 ranibizumab/bevacizumab

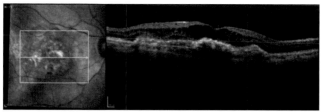

Figure 8-1. OCT showing persistent intraretinal fluid 1 month after receiving 50 monthly bevacizumab injections. Visual acuity was 20/60. The left panel shows an infrared reflectance image of the fundus.

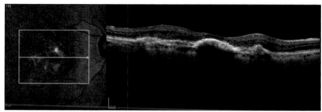

Figure 8-2. OCT of patient in Figure 8-1 1 month after the first aflibercept injection shows dramatic improvement in intraretinal fluid, with a visual acuity of 20/50. The left panel shows an infrared reflectance image of the fundus.

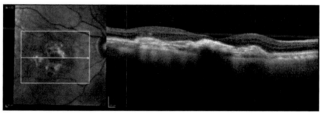

Figure 8-3. OCT of patient in Figure 8-1 1 month after the second aflibercept injection shows complete resolution of intraretinal fluid, with 20/40 visual acuity. The left panel shows an infrared reflectance image of the fundus.

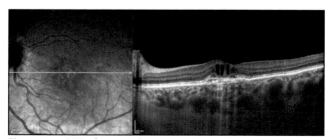

Figure 8-4. OCT of a second patient with persistent intraretinal fluid after 11 monthly injections of ranibizumab. Visual acuity was 20/200. The decision was made at this visit to switch to aflibercept. The left panel shows an infrared reflectance image of the fundus.

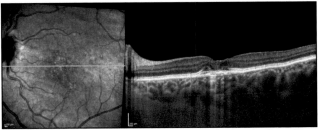

Figure 8-5. OCT of patient in Figure 8-4 1 month after the first afliber-cept injection shows resolution of the intraretinal fluid. Visual acuity remained 20/200. The left panel shows an infrared reflectance image of the fundus.

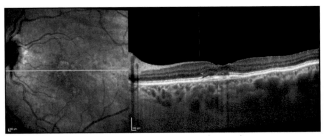

Figure 8-6. OCT of patient in Figure 8-4 shows that response was maintained after 4 more aflibercept injections. The left panel shows an infrared reflectance image of the fundus.

injections.[10] After an average of 4.4 aflibercept injections over 6 months, 64% of eyes showed an anatomical improvement, without an improvement in visual acuity.[10]

A group in New York evaluated 34 eyes with persistent fluid after an average of 28.6 ranibizumab injections and reported improvement in both anatomy and visual acuity at 6 months on aflibercept treatment.[13] Anatomically, there was improvement in central foveal thickness, as well as pigment epithelial detachment height and diameter, and visual acuity improved from 20/75 to 20/60.[13]

INCREASED ANTI-VASCULAR ENDOTHELIAL GROWTH FACTOR DOSING

Perhaps the best evidence on AMD treatment failures comes from the Super-Dose Anti-VEGF trial.[14,15] This study enrolled 87 patients with recalcitrant disease, defined as persistent leakage on fluorescein angiography or spectral-domain OCT despite a mean of 24 monthly injections. These patients were given a quadruple dose (2.0 mg) of ranibi-zumab monthly for 3 months, followed by monthly pro re nata (PRN) quadruple doses for 19 months, which achieved a statistically significant mean gain of 3.6 letters of Early Treatment Diabetic Retinopathy Study (ETDRS) acuity. Interestingly, this type of benefit ascribed to high-dose ranibizumab was not detected in the HARBOR study (Phase III, Double-Masked, Multicenter, Randomized, Active Treatment-Controlled Study of the Efficacy and Safety of 0.5 mg and 2.0 mg Ranibizumab Administered Monthly or on an As-Needed Basis [PRN] in Patients With Subfoveal Neovascular Age-Related Macular

Degeneration), which compared newly diagnosed wet AMD patients taking either 0.5 or 2.0 mg ranibizumab.[16] Importantly, the HARBOR study was designed to evaluate the efficacy of high-dose therapy in treatment-naïve patients, not recalcitrant AMD; therefore, the negative finding of super-dose ranibizumab in the HARBOR study cannot be directly extrapolated to suboptimal responders. Ranibizumab 2.0 mg currently remains unavailable for use.

Another strategy for increasing the frequency of anti-VEGF injections was reported by Stewart et al.[17] Following a report from a dose- and frequency-ranging phase II study of ranibizumab,[18] the investigators used mathematical modeling based on the time-dependent relative binding activities of bevacizumab, ranibizumab, and aflibercept. The simulation found an improved pharmacokinetic profile with short-term biweekly dosing. The investigators also modeled increasing the dose of various agents and predicted that biweekly, standard-dose bevacizumab would produce higher trough levels than a quadruple dose of ranibizumab monthly. Of note, low-dose (0.5 mg) aflibercept produced trough binding activities 32 to 134 times higher than those for biweekly, standard-dose bevacizumab in this simulation, suggesting that the use of aflibercept may obviate the need for increased treatment frequency.

COMBINATION THERAPY

Although not specifically targeted to the treatment failure patient population, there are several reports of combining anti-VEGF therapy with other treatment modalities in treatment-naïve patients. The DENALI study compared monthly ranibizumab with either full- or reduced-fluence verteporfin photodynamic therapy (PDT), combined with a PRN regimen of ranibizumab in 321 treatment-naïve patients.[19] After 1 year, results in the 2 combination therapy groups did not meet the predetermined noninferiority limit of 7 ETDRS letters. In fact, there was a trend for less of an improvement in the combined therapy groups compared with monotherapy. Likewise, improvement in central retinal thickness was less in the PDT groups. Due to the fact that the monotherapy group received monthly therapy (mean 7.6 injections following the initial 3 doses), and the PDT groups received PRN therapy (2.2 and 2.8 injections following the initial 3 doses), it is difficult to discern how the difference in anti-VEGF regimens is responsible for the visual and anatomical outcomes.

A companion to the DENALI study was the MONT BLANC trial, in which 255 treatment-naïve patients were randomized to receive standard-fluence PDT combined with PRN ranibizumab or PRN ranibizumab monotherapy.[20] In this study, the mean change in visual acuity was similarly low in the 2 groups after 12 months, with mean improvement of 4.4 ETDRS letters in the monotherapy group and 2.5 letters in the combination therapy group.[20] Importantly, there was not a significant difference in the number of injections received in either arm (1.9 in the combination group vs 2.2 in the monotherapy group after 3 loading doses), suggesting that the addition of PDT did not allow for a reduction of anti-VEGF injections.

Several investigators have reported the use of triple therapy, combining anti-VEGF therapy, PDT, and intravitreal or sub-Tenon's corticosteroids. In one retrospective study of 31 eyes, patients received bevacizumab, low-fluence PDT, and posterior sub-Tenon's triamcinolone, with retreatment on a PRN basis.[21] After 6-month follow-up, there was a 9-letter improvement in visual acuity and an improvement in central retinal thickness on OCT of 87.7 μm.[21] In another retrospective analysis, 61 treatment-naïve eyes received either bevacizumab or ranibizumab, combined with intravitreal dexamethasone and full-fluence PDT.[22] This cohort was compared with 40 eyes that received anti-VEGF monotherapy. Both groups experienced a significant improvement in visual acuity, but the triple-therapy group received significantly fewer injections (1.9 vs 3.1) over 14 months of follow-up.[22] The applicability of these results to treatment failures is unknown, but these studies provide proof-of-concept to support trying this modality in select cases.

CATEGORIES OF TREATMENT FAILURES

There has been much debate as to what constitutes a treatment failure, but, in general, patients can be subdivided into several categories. Some patients fail to demonstrate a favorable response from the outset and may truly be considered nonresponders. Other individuals exhibit an initial expected visual and anatomic response but then experience a plateau with persistent but stable fluid, particularly in the subretinal and sub-RPE locations. This type of response might be considered an incomplete responder. Such incomplete response is consistent with good visual outcome in many eyes. Other patients demonstrate an initial complete cessation of exudation followed late by recurrence, despite continued therapy. These patients could be considered resistant, tolerant, or possibly exhibiting tachyphylaxis, depending on the specifics of their dosing strategy and treatment response.

In the case of a nonresponder, an important initial step is to verify the diagnosis. As discussed in Chapter 5, there are several common mimickers of wet AMD that do not respond well to anti-VEGF therapy. We recommend early consideration of repeat fluorescein angiography, indocyanine green angiography, fundus autofluorescence, high-resolution (spectral-domain) OCT, careful elicitation of medication history to identify any possible corticosteroid exposure, and other investigations based on the clinical situation. It is important to remember that in the ANCHOR, MARINA, and VIEW 1 and 2 studies, the mean improvement in visual acuity was rapid, with much less visual acuity gain after the first 3 injections.

In wet AMD patients who are nonresponsive or suboptimally responsive to a particular medication, consider switching agents as a first tactic, followed by biweekly injections if the response is suboptimal. Before increasing dosing frequency, it may be helpful to evaluate the patient at a 1- or 2-week interval after an anti-VEGF injection, to assess whether the medication had an initial effect that then wore off by the 4-week visit. Such patients might also be able to give a history of improvement that peaks and then diminishes during the follow-up interval. If using aflibercept, although the VIEW trials showed similar anatomic and visual outcomes in eyes treated with aflibercept every 4 weeks compared with those treated every 8 weeks after an initial loading dose, incomplete responders might require monthly aflibercept to maintain anatomic and visual gains. Finally, there may be a role for combining anti-VEGF injection with PDT, thermal laser, and/or corticosteroids in such patients.

Patients who develop tolerance can be the most vexing because they exhibit a complete response after the initial treatment but then lose ground while on the same previously successful regimen. Practically speaking, such patients may have been receiving less than monthly injections when they become tolerant. Many clinicians will attempt to space out injections in a complete responder, in either a PRN or treat-and-extend fashion. Any patient receiving less than monthly therapy with a significant recurrence should have their treatment interval shortened. Patients in whom treatment has rapidly lost effectiveness may have developed tachyphylaxis. In these patients, stopping therapy briefly may restore a good response to the initial anti-VEGF agent; they may also respond to switching agents. For patients who have slowly developed tolerance, increasing the drug frequency or switching agents may be the most efficacious step.

SUMMARY

We now have the luxury of using 3 highly effective anti-VEGF agents to treat wet AMD. However, patients who have no response, incomplete response, or recurrent disease, despite good adherence to standard dosing regimens, can be challenging. Ultimately, the clinician has only 3 real options: switch the anti-VEGF agent, increase the dosage or frequency of therapy, or combine the anti-VEGF injection with another modality, such as PDT. Unfortunately, there is no conclusive evidence to guide clinicians, but defining the nature of a given patient's treatment failure may help to guide a therapeutic approach, and future studies focusing on this population may help to devise treatment algorithms for these difficult-to-manage patients.

REFERENCES

1. Rosenfeld PJ, Brown DM, Heier JS, et al. Ranibizumab for neovascular age-related macular degeneration. *N Engl J Med*. 2006;355:1419-1431.
2. Brown DM, Michels M, Kaiser PK, et al. Ranibizumab versus verteporfin photodynamic therapy for neovascular age-related macular degeneration: two-year results of the ANCHOR study. *Ophthalmology*. 2009;116:57-65.e5.
3. Heier JS, Brown DM, Chong V, et al. Intravitreal aflibercept (VEGF trap-eye) in wet age-related macular degeneration. *Ophthalmology*. 2012;119:2537-2548.
4. Group CR, Martin DF, Maguire MG, et al. Ranibizumab and bevacizumab for neovascular age-related macular degeneration. *N Engl J Med*. 2011;364:1897-1908.
5. Eghoj MS, Sorensen TL. Tachyphylaxis during treatment of exudative age-related macular degeneration with ranibizumab. *Br J Ophthalmol*. 2012;96:21-23.
6. Gasperini JL, Fawzi AA, Khondkaryan A, et al. Bevacizumab and ranibizumab tachyphylaxis in the treatment of choroidal neovascularisation. *Br J Ophthalmol*. 2012;96:14-20.
7. Bakall B, Folk JC, Boldt HC, et al. Aflibercept therapy for exudative age-related macular degeneration resistant to bevacizumab and ranibizumab. *Am J Ophthalmol*. 2013;156:15-22.e1.
8. Ho VY, Yeh S, Olsen TW, et al. Short-term outcomes of aflibercept for neovascular age-related macular degeneration in eyes previously treated with other vascular endothelial growth factor inhibitors. *Am J Ophthalmol*. 2013;156:23-28.e2.
9. Yonekawa Y, Andreoli C, Miller JB, et al. Conversion to aflibercept for chronic refractory or recurrent neovascular age-related macular degeneration. *Am J Ophthalmol*. 2013;156:29-35.e2.
10. Cho H, Shah CP, Weber M, Heier JS. Aflibercept for exudative AMD with persistent fluid on ranibizumab and/or bevacizumab. *Br J Ophthalmol*. 2013;97:1032-1035.
11. Patel KH, Chow CC, Rathod R, et al. Rapid response of retinal pigment epithelial detachments to intravitreal aflibercept in neovascular age-related macular degeneration refractory to bevacizumab and ranibizumab. *Eye (Lond)*. 2013;27:663-667.
12. Schachat AP. Switching anti-vascular endothelial growth factor therapy for neovascular age-related macular degeneration. *Am J Ophthalmol*. 2013;156:1-2.e1.
13. Kumar N, Marsiglia M, Mrejen S, et al. Visual and anatomical outcomes of intravitreal aflibercept in eyes with persistent subfoveal fluid despite previous treatments with ranibizumab in patients with neovascular age-related macular degeneration. *Retina*. 2013;33(8):1605-1612.

14. Brown DM, Chen E, Mariani A, Major JC Jr. Super-dose anti-VEGF (SAVE) trial: 2.0 mg intravitreal ranibizumab for recalcitrant neovascular macular degeneration-primary end point. *Ophthalmology.* 2013;120:349-354.

15. Wykoff CC, Brown DM, Croft DE, Wong TP. Two year SAVE outcomes: 2.0 mg ranibizumab for recalcitrant neovascular AMD. *Ophthalmology.* 2013;120:1945-1946.e1.

16. Busbee BG, Ho AC, Brown DM, et al. Twelve-month efficacy and safety of 0.5 mg or 2.0 mg ranibizumab in patients with subfoveal neovascular age-related macular degeneration. *Ophthalmology.* 2013;120:1046-1056.

17. Stewart MW, Rosenfeld PJ, Penha FM, et al. Pharmacokinetic rationale for dosing every 2 weeks versus 4 weeks with intravitreal ranibizumab, bevacizumab, and aflibercept (vascular endothelial growth factor Trap-eye). *Retina.* 2012;32(3):434-457.

18. Rosenfeld PJ, Heier JS, Hantsbarger G, Shams N. Tolerability and efficacy of multiple escalating doses of ranibizumab (Lucentis) for neovascular age-related macular degeneration. *Ophthalmology.* 2006;113:623.e1

19. Kaiser PK, Boyer DS, Cruess AF, Slakter JS, Pilz S, Weisberger A. Verteporfin plus ranibizumab for choroidal neovascularization in age-related macular degeneration: twelve-month results of the DENALI study. *Ophthalmology.* 2012;119:1001-1010.

20. Larsen M, Schmidt-Erfurth U, Lanzetta P, et al. Verteporfin plus ranibizumab for choroidal neovascularization in age-related macular degeneration: twelve-month MONT BLANC study results. *Ophthalmology.* 2012;119:992-1000.

21. Kovacs KD, Quirk MT, Kinoshita T, et al. A retrospective analysis of triple combination therapy with intravitreal bevacizumab, posterior sub-tenon's triamcinolone acetonide, and low-fluence verteporfin photodynamic therapy in patients with neovascular age-related macular degeneration. *Retina.* 2011;31:446-452.

22. Forte R, Bonavolonta P, Benayoun Y, Adenis JP, Robert PY. Intravitreal ranibizumab and bevacizumab in combination with full-fluence verteporfin therapy and dexamethasone for exudative age-related macular degeneration. *Ophthalmic Res.* 2011;45:129-134.

9

SURGERY FOR AGE-RELATED MACULAR DEGENERATION

Christopher J. Brady, MD and Carl D. Regillo, MD

Neovascular (wet) age-related macular degeneration (AMD) is a primarily medically managed disease. As discussed in previous chapters, there are currently 3 highly effective intravitreal anti-vascular endothelial growth factor (anti-VEGF) inhibitors to treat nearly all cases of acute wet AMD. In addition, photodynamic therapy (PDT) and laser photocoagulation are also available, which may be useful in certain select cases of wet AMD, usually in combination with anti-VEGF therapy. However, circumstances exist when AMD becomes potentially amenable to a surgical approach, most notably in the management of large submacular hemorrhages. Other attempts have been made in the past to surgically manage wet AMD, but these approaches are now primarily of historical interest. These approaches include the surgical removal of choroidal neovascularization (CNV), macular translocation, and intraocular radiotherapy.

SURGICAL REMOVAL OF CHOROIDAL NEOVASCULARIZATION

In a 1988 report, de Juan and Machemer[1] described a technique for pars plana vitrectomy (PPV) and submacular scar removal, with encouraging results in several cases. In 1991, Blinder et al[2] reported a technique that also included transplantation of the retinal pigment epithelium (RPE).[2] The basic technique was to perform a standard 3-port PPV, followed by large circumferential retinotomy around the macula. The neurosensory retina was then reflected, and the exposed CNV was removed. Refinements of the technique were published in the early 1990s,[3] which recommended creation of a small posterior retinotomy with optional infusion of balanced salt solution (BSS) to create a small subretinal bleb. The CNV complex was mobilized with an angulated pick and then grasped and removed with angulated forceps. Soon afterward, a large prospective study, called the Submacular Surgery Trial (SST), was designed to evaluate the potential benefits of the surgical removal of CNV in patients with wet AMD; 454 patients with wet AMD without submacular blood and 336 patients with submacular blood were included.[4] Participants were randomized to submacular surgery or observation groups. CNV

Duker JS, Witkin AJ, eds.
*Age-Related Macular Degeneration:
Current Management (pp. 129-137)*
© 2015 Taylor & Francis Group

removal surgery was the subject of a Cochrane Database systematic review published in 2009.[5] This review included 2 reports from the SST and concluded that there was high-quality evidence that indicated this surgery does not prevent vision loss compared with observation. They also noted an increased risk of cataract and retinal detachment following submacular surgery for the removal of CNV. Therefore, this type of submacular surgery is now rarely performed for CNV secondary to AMD.

MACULAR TRANSLOCATION SURGERY

A novel surgical approach to treat vision loss in AMD was described by Machemer and Steinhorst[6] in 1993 in an animal model. The procedure involved PPV with injection of subretinal BSS to deliberately detach the macula, followed by repositioning of the macula to a new location with healthier underlying RPE tissue. Initial reports by Machemer and Steinhorst[7] also described inducing a complete serous retinal detachment with BSS, making a large peripheral circumferential retinotomy, rotating the retina and relocating the macula, adhering the retina with laser, and, finally, silicone oil tamponade. A limited macular translocation was subsequently described,[8] which involved detachment of the temporal retina, followed by arcuate shortening of the choroid and sclera parallel to the limbus. This technique creates a limited lateral translocation of the macula, without the need for a large peripheral retinectomy.

A Cochrane Database systematic review of macular translocation was published in 2008.[9] A single randomized, controlled trial of 50 eyes of 50 patients was identified in the search.[10] In this trial, participants were randomized to macular translocation or PDT and were followed for 12 months. Several visual acuity outcomes were analyzed. Ten (40%) of 25 translocation patients experienced a gain of 3 or more lines of Early Treatment Diabetic Retinopathy Study (ETDRS) visual acuity. The mean change in visual acuity was a gain of 2.7 letters in the translocation arm vs a loss of 11.9 letters in the PDT arm of the study. However, the authors concluded that the evidence generated by this small trial was not sufficient to recommend translocation, particularly in light of the reported significant complications, which included retinal detachment with proliferative vitreoretinopathy, high rate of CNV recurrence, and the frequent need for eye muscle surgery following macular translocation.

SURGICAL RADIATION THERAPY

Because CNV is caused by an abnormal proliferation of vascular tissue, the idea of applying radiation therapy to inhibit endothelial cell proliferation is logical and has been attempted by several groups. Original attempts to treat wet AMD with external radiation were not found to be effective.[11] In an attempt to improve efficacy, more focal radiation delivery systems were developed, one of which was a strontium probe that was held over the macula during PPV. This approach, referred to as epiretinal macular brachytherapy (EMBT), was tested in several prospective clinical studies, including the published the CNV Secondary to AMD Treated With Beta Radiation Epiretinal Therapy (CABERNET)[12] and Macular Epiretinal Brachytherapy in Treated Age-Related Macular Degeneration (MERITAGE)[13] trials. The CABERNET study enrolled 494 patients with treatment-naïve exudative AMD who were randomized to receive either EMBT with 2 monthly doses of ranibizumab or as-needed ranibizumab with a minimum of quarterly maintenance dosing; patients were followed for 2 years. The EMBT treatment was applied for approximately 4 minutes through a 20-gauge pars plana incision as part of a standard 3-port PPV. After 24 months, 77% of the EMBT group and 90% of the control group lost fewer than 15 letters of ETDRS acuity. Because the prespecified, noninferiority margin was 10%, the authors concluded that the study did not support routine use of EMBT in this population.

The MERITAGE study[13] was a prospective, noncontrolled trial of 53 eyes in 53 patients with wet AMD who required frequent anti-VEGF treatments. All participants received EMBT as well as ranibizumab as needed at monthly intervals per predefined retreatment criteria, and they were followed for 12 months. At the end of follow-up, the mean change in vision was a loss of 4 ETDRS letters, and the mean change in central retinal thickness on optical coherence tomography (OCT) increased by 50 μm. Importantly, participants required a mean of 3.49 anti-VEGF injections in the follow-up period. The authors concluded that EMBT may provide a means to reduce the frequency of injections for those patients who require frequent anti-VEGF retreatment; however, there was no comparison arm in the study. This radiation delivery system is not US Food and Drug Administration approved, and it is not available in the United States.

SURGERY FOR SUBMACULAR HEMORRHAGE

A large hemorrhage under the macula is one of the dreaded complications of wet AMD. Patients with large submacular hemorrhages have a poor visual prognosis. Most patients present with poor vision, which then worsens in up to 80% of cases without treatment.[14] Despite the success of anti-VEGF therapy for wet AMD, the optimal management of submacular hemorrhages associated with AMD remains poorly defined.[15,16] This is due in part to the exclusion of patients with large submacular hemorrhages from the major pivotal trials testing various anti-VEGF therapeutics for wet AMD. The SST provides some information on the surgical management of submacular hemorrhage[4]; however, most of the techniques used in these trials are now outdated. Further guidance about submacular hemorrhage is limited to smaller, uncontrolled series.[17]

Over the years, various small series suggest more promising results by using an intravitreal gas bubble, with or without PPV and with or without tissue plasminogen activator (tPA), to displace submacular hemorrhage away from the macula. The decision to manage AMD-related submacular hemorrhages with a displacement procedure is based on the location, size, and thickness of the hemorrhage. Patients with small, thin submacular hemorrhages mostly outside the foveal center are best managed by anti-VEGF therapy alone. Patients with larger hemorrhages (more than 6 disc areas) that are relatively thick and centered in the macula may be considered for a pneumatic displacement procedure, especially if the hemorrhage is less than 3 weeks in duration and if the patient had reasonably good vision before the hemorrhage. Displacing a submacular hemorrhage can be done in the office with an intravitreal injection of an expansile gas (with or without an intravitreal injection of tPA) or in the operating room with a PPV, subretinal tPA injection, and fluid-gas exchange (Figures 9-1 to 9-3).[17-19] We believe that the surgical approach described in this chapter produces a more reliable, complete displacement of the submacular hemorrhage away from the macula, and it is usually our preferred technique.

A history of poor visual acuity prior to submacular hemorrhage development is a relative contraindication to surgical intervention. Patients with massive subretinal hemorrhages that extend significantly into the peripheral retina may not be good candidates

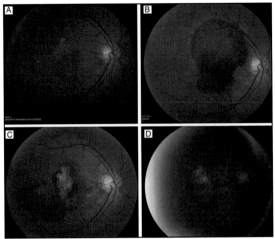

Figure 9-1. Color fundus photographs of Case 1. (A) Eighteen months prior to submacular hemorrhage, CNV was noted in the subfoveal region and anti-VEGF therapy was initiated. Visual acuity was 20/80. (B) Acute submacular hemorrhage occurred during the course of anti-VEGF therapy, and visual acuity declined to 20/400. (C) Two months after pars plana vitrectomy and subretinal tPA, the subretinal hemorrhage was much thinner. (D) One year postoperatively, there was some increased atrophy but no hemorrhage or fibrosis, and vision improved to 20/200.

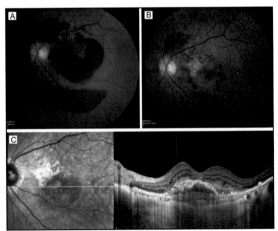

Figure 9-2. Case 2. (A) Color fundus photograph of a patient who presented with an acute submacular hemorrhage due to AMD and decreased visual acuity to counting fingers. One month prior, visual acuity was 20/50. (B) Color fundus photograph 1 month after pars plana vitrectomy and subretinal tPA. The hemorrhage was partially displaced, and mild subretinal fibrosis was present. (C) Three months postoperatively, spectral-domain OCT with infrared reflectance image (left panel) showed central subretinal fibrosis. The patient's vision remained poor in the counting fingers range with only minimal subjective visual improvement.

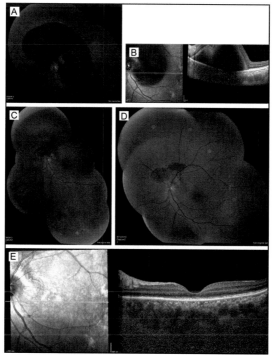

Figure 9-3. Case 3. (A) Color fundus photograph of acute submacular hemorrhage due to polypoidal choroidal vasculopathy with a presenting visual acuity of counting fingers. (B) Corresponding spectral-domain OCT with infrared reflectance image (left panel) showed a large amount of subretinal hyper-reflectivity consistent with blood. (C) Color fundus photograph 3 weeks after pars plana vitrectomy showed excellent displacement of subretinal hemorrhage from the macula. (D) Color fundus photograph 2 months postoperatively showed only a small amount of residual subretinal hemorrhage outside the macula, and visual acuity improved to 20/25. (E) Spectral-domain OCT with infrared reflectance image (left panel) 2 months postoperatively showed only minor outer retinal distortion but no central subretinal fibrosis or neovascularization. In this case, the polypoidal neovascularization was located in the superior peripapillary region.

for hemorrhage displacement. Large RPE detachments are a relative contraindication to surgical displacement. If the decision is made to proceed with surgery, perioperative anti-VEGF therapy should still be performed on a regular treatment schedule.

Surgical Technique

The 2 main modalities for the PPV/tPA displacement technique to treat submacular hemorrhage are pharmacological and mechanical. The tissue plasminogen activator is a 70-kDa recombinant human protein that cleaves native plasminogen into plasmin. Plasmin is an enzyme that breaks down fibrin, which is a principal component of clotted

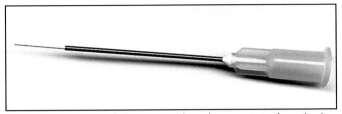

Figure 9-4. Microcannula (41-gauge tip) used to penetrate the retina in a self-sealing manner to infuse tPA in the subretinal space during the vitrectomy displacement procedure.

blood, within minutes of direct contact. The molecule is principally used as a thrombolytic in the setting of nonhemorrhagic acute stroke, but it is used off-label for many purposes throughout medicine. After injection of tPA into the subretinal space and its enzymatic lysis of fibrin within the clot, the hemorrhage is then amenable to displacement. In large hemorrhages secondary to wet AMD, the enzymatic lysis and pneumatic displacement procedure is thought to provide a gentler reapposition of the neurosensory retina and RPE than a purely mechanical evacuation of hemorrhage.[20]

After a standard core PPV (with separation of the posterior hyaloid if attached to the posterior pole), a 39- or 41-gauge needle (Figure 9-4) is used to inject tPA (25 or 50 mcg/0.1 mL) directly into the submacular space. This small-sized catheter allows for injection of fluid into the subretinal space through a tiny, self-sealing retinotomy, which is usually made superior to the horizontal meridian so that it may be more easily tamponaded by the gas. A generous bleb of subretinal fluid that extends beyond the borders of the submacular hemorrhage appears to maximize the postoperative displacement. Note that with the current surgical displacement approach, there is no attempt to evacuate the subretinal blood directly or to remove the neovascular complex. A 75% to 100% fluid-air exchange is then performed. The air may, in turn, be exchanged with 20% to 25% SF6 gas if a longer-lasting tamponade is desired.

Patients typically are instructed to maintain face-forward positioning for 24 to 48 hours. Some surgeons recommend a face-down position, whereas others do not feel strict positioning is necessary and recommend keeping the head upright to displace the hemorrhage inferiorly.

Variations in Technique

Numerous variations of the surgical technique have been reported. Some are of historic interest but are illustrative of the evolution of the management of this condition. Initially, surgeons attempted mechanical evacuation of the submacular hemorrhage/CNV complex.[4] This technique required creation of a large posterior retinotomy and aspiration of the clot. The entire CNV complex was then grasped with submacular forceps and removed through the retinotomy. The complex was sometimes segmented if it was too large to be removed en bloc. The retinotomy was sealed with endolaser photocoagulation only if it was larger than 1 disc diameter. This technique was used in the SST prior to the introduction of small 39- or 41-gauge translocation cannulas, which are now used to inject subretinal tPA.[16] Other surgeons have reported use of preoperative intravitreal tPA 24 hours prior to PPV with use of heavy liquid (perfluoron) and peripheral retinotomy to drain the submacular hemorrhage.[16] Surgeons in Japan have described this technique, where the majority of the included population had polypoidal choroidal vasculopathy (PCV), but their results may not be applicable to all patients with wet AMD. Conversely, many patients with PCV may respond to a standard PPV/tPA displacement approach as described previously (see Figure 9-3).

Various techniques of subretinal tPA injection exist. Some surgeons create an initial subretinal bleb with one or more injections of BSS to dilute the submacular hemorrhage and fully detach the macula, followed by injection of concentrated tPA into the bleb. Fluorescein dye can be added to the tPA solution to allow for better visualization of the tPA. Some surgeons advocate intraoperative anti-VEGF therapy, either into the vitreous cavity or subretinally. Some surgeons are now injecting an air bubble into the clot subretinally to help facilitate postoperative blood displacement.[21]

Complications

Postoperative retinal tears, retinal detachment, and proliferative vitreoretinopathy are potential complications of submacular hemorrhage displacement. These complications were more common with older surgical approaches, which used large retinotomies to directly evacuate the hemorrhage. Vitreous hemorrhage, macular hole, recurrent submacular hemorrhage, and RPE tear formation have all been reported following PPV with tPA for submacular hemorrhage displacement.[19,22] PPV accelerates cataract progression, and there may be an increased risk of open-angle glaucoma following PPV. Endophthalmitis is a potential rare complication of any intraocular procedure.

Tissue plasminogen activator may have theoretical retinal or RPE toxicity. All patients in one series who received 100 μg intravitreal tPA were diagnosed with inferior exudative retinal detachment following injection.[23] None of the patients who received a 50-μg dose experienced this. It is unclear what the mechanism was for this exudative response.

Surgical Outcomes

Level I evidence supporting the efficacy of any intervention for AMD-related large submacular hemorrhage is not available, but because the natural history is poor, any evidence suggesting a favorable effect compared with the natural history is encouraging.[20] Most series that used small needles or microcannulas to create a self-sealing retinotomy using the technique described previously have reported mean improvements in vision postoperatively; one series reported visual improvement in 73% (8 of 11) eyes, with a mean follow-up of 6.5 months.[24] Olivier et al[25] reported 2 or more lines of vision gained in 68% (17 of 25) of eyes at 3-month follow-up. Sandhu et al[26] reported 83% of 16 patients reaching the same 2-or-more-line improvement endpoint at 6 months. In a larger, more recent retrospective case series, Chang et al[19] reported that 82% of 101 eyes had at least one line of improvement in postoperative acuity at 3 months.

SUMMARY

Several surgical approaches have been developed to address the complications of wet AMD. Submacular CNV excision surgery and macular translocation have not been shown to have significant visual benefit compared with the high rates of postoperative complications and have since largely been abandoned and replaced with anti-VEGF treatments of wet AMD. The role of surgically delivered brachytherapy has also been explored, with disappointing results in phase III testing. Although generally devastating, submacular hemorrhage seems to be the complication of AMD that is most amenable to surgical intervention. High-quality evidence supporting the optimal treatment strategy is lacking, so clinicians must rely on various published case series to develop a management plan for each patient. Duration, location, size, and thickness of the hemorrhage are factors used to determine whether a displacement intervention should be considered in addition to anti-VEGF therapy. PPV with subretinal tPA and gas tamponade can be a good option for patients with recent moderate- to large-sized, thick central hemorrhages if there is known to be limited preexisting damage from AMD.

REFERENCES

1. de Juan E Jr, Machemer R. Vitreous surgery for hemorrhagic and fibrous complications of age-related macular degeneration. *Am J Ophthalmol.* 1988;105:25-29.
2. Blinder KJ, Peyman GA, Paris CL, Gremillion CM Jr. Submacular scar excision in age-related macular degeneration. *Int Ophthalmol.* 1991;15:215-222.
3. Lambert HM, Capone A Jr, Aaberg TM, Sternberg P Jr, Mandell BA, Lopez PF. Surgical excision of subfoveal neovascular membranes in age-related macular degeneration. *Am J Ophthalmol.* 1992;113:257-262.
4. Bressler NM, Bressler SB, Childs AL, et al. Surgery for hemorrhagic choroidal neovascular lesions of age-related macular degeneration: ophthalmic findings: SST report no. 13. *Ophthalmology.* 2004;111:1993-2006.
5. Giansanti F, Eandi CM, Virgili G. Submacular surgery for choroidal neovascularisation secondary to age-related macular degeneration. *Cochrane Database Syst Rev.* 2009;2:CD006931.
6. Machemer R, Steinhorst UH. Retinal separation, retinotomy, and macular relocation: I. Experimental studies in the rabbit eye. *Graefes Arch Clin Exp Ophthalmol.* 1993;231:629-634.
7. Machemer R, Steinhorst UH. Retinal separation, retinotomy, and macular relocation: II. A surgical approach for age-related macular degeneration? *Graefes Arch Clin Exp Ophthalmol.* 1993;231:635-641.
8. de Juan E Jr, Loewenstein A, Bressler NM, Alexander J. Translocation of the retina for management of subfoveal choroidal neovascularization II: a preliminary report in humans. *Am J Ophthalmol.* 1998;125:635-646.
9. Eandi CM, Giansanti F, Virgili G. Macular translocation for neovascular age-related macular degeneration. *Cochrane Database Syst Rev.* 2008;4:CD006928.
10. Gelisken F, Voelker M, Schwabe R, et al. Full macular translocation versus photodynamic therapy with verteporfin in the treatment of neovascular age-related macular degeneration: 1-year results of a prospective, controlled, randomised pilot trial (FMT-PDT). *Graefes Arch Clin Exp Ophthalmol.* 2007;245:1085-1095.
11. Evans JR, Sivagnanavel V, Chong V. Radiotherapy for neovascular age-related macular degeneration. *Cochrane Database Syst Rev.* 2010;5:CD004004.
12. Dugel PU, Bebchuk JD, Nau J, et al. Epimacular brachytherapy for neovascular age-related macular degeneration: a randomized, controlled trial (CABERNET). *Ophthalmology.* 2013;120:317-327.
13. Dugel PU, Petrarca R, Bennett M, et al. Macular epiretinal brachytherapy in treated age-related macular degeneration: MERITAGE study: twelve-month safety and efficacy results. *Ophthalmology.* 2012;119:1425-1431.
14. Scupola A, Coscas G, Soubrane G, Balestrazzi E. Natural history of macular subretinal hemorrhage in age-related macular degeneration. *Ophthalmologica.* 1999;213:97-102.
15. Tennant MT, Borrillo JL, Regillo CD. Management of submacular hemorrhage. *Ophthalmol Clin North Am.* 2002;15:445-452.
16. Steel DH, Sandhu SS. Submacular haemorrhages associated with neovascular age-related macular degeneration. *Br J Ophthalmol.* 2011;95:1051-1057.
17. Shultz RW, Bakri SJ. Treatment for submacular hemorrhage associated with neovascular age-related macular degeneration. *Semin Ophthalmol.* 2011;26:361-371.

18. Hassan AS, Johnson MW, Schneiderman TE, et al. Management of submacular hemorrhage with intravitreous tissue plasminogen activator injection and pneumatic displacement. *Ophthalmology.* 1999;106:1900-1906.

19. Chang W, Garg SJ, Maturi R, et al. Management of thick submacular hemorrhage with subretinal tissue plasminogen activator and pneumatic displacement for age-related macular degeneration. *Am J Ophthalmol.* 2014;157:1250-1257.

20. van Zeeburg EJ, van Meurs JC. Literature review of recombinant tissue plasminogen activator used for recent-onset submacular hemorrhage displacement in age-related macular degeneration. *Ophthalmologica.* 2013;229:1-14.

21. Martel JN, Mahmoud TH. Subretinal pneumatic displacement of subretinal hemorrhage. *JAMA Ophthalmol.* 2013;131:1632-1635.

22. Fine HF, Iranmanesh R, Del Priore LV, et al. Surgical outcomes after massive subretinal hemorrhage secondary to age-related macular degeneration. *Retina.* 2010;30:1588-1594.

23. Hesse L, Schmidt J, Kroll P. Management of acute submacular hemorrhage using recombinant tissue plasminogen activator and gas. *Graefes Arch Clin Exp Ophthalmol.* 1999;237:273-277.

24. Haupert CL, McCuen BW II, Jaffe GJ, et al. Pars plana vitrectomy, subretinal injection of tissue plasminogen activator, and fluid-gas exchange for displacement of thick submacular hemorrhage in age-related macular degeneration. *Am J Ophthalmol.* 2001;131:208-215.

25. Olivier S, Chow DR, Packo KH, MacCumber MW, Awh CC. Subretinal recombinant tissue plasminogen activator injection and pneumatic displacement of thick submacular hemorrhage in Age-Related macular degeneration. *Ophthalmology.* 2004;111:1201-1208.

26. Sandhu SS, Manvikar S, Steel DH. Displacement of submacular hemorrhage associated with age-related macular degeneration using vitrectomy and submacular tPA injection followed by intravitreal ranibizumab. *Clin Ophthalmol.* 2010;4:637-642.

10

FUTURE THERAPIES

Roger A. Goldberg, MD, MBA and Jeffrey S. Heier, MD

Despite monumental advances in therapy over the past decade, age-related macular degeneration (AMD) remains the most common cause of visual impairment in the developed world.[1-3] Given the huge disease burden of AMD and the success of currently available therapies such as US Food and Drug Administration-approved ranibizumab and aflibercept, as well as off-label bevacizumab, considerable resources are being deployed to develop new treatments for both the neovascular (wet) and non-neovascular (dry) forms of AMD. Treatment goals for wet AMD are to improve visual outcomes and decrease the burden of frequent intravitreal injections, which are often required with today's vascular endothelial growth factor (VEGF) inhibitors. In geographic atrophy (GA), a disease for which no therapies are currently available, the goals are more basic: slow or stop disease progression. Ultimately, the ideal therapies for AMD will identify those patients at risk for vision loss and treat them before one of the advanced forms of AMD manifests itself.

For both patients and clinicians alike, this is an exciting time in the research and development of new AMD therapies. A broad set of disease pathways and drug delivery methods are being studied to develop the next generation of therapies for both wet and dry AMD, and, over the next decade, retina specialists hope to have many additional options to treat—and perhaps prevent—vision loss associated with AMD.

ANTIANGIOGENIC AGENTS

Many studies, and now years of clinical experience, have proven the efficacy of VEGF inhibitors in wet AMD. The ANCHOR (Anti-Vascular Endothelial Growth Factor Antibody for the Treatment of Predominantly Classic CNV in AMD)[4] and MARINA (Minimally Classic/Occult Trial of the Anti-Vascular Endothelial Growth Factor Antibody Ranibizumab in the Treatment of Neovascular AMD)[5] trials paved the way for the approval of ranibizumab, and, although it had been used off-label since 2006, the CATT (Comparison of AMD Treatment Trials) study showed equivalent efficacy of bevacizumab compared with ranibizumab in the treatment of wet AMD.[6] In all of these

Duker JS, Witkin AJ, eds.
*Age-Related Macular Degeneration:
Current Management (pp. 139-145)*
© 2015 Taylor & Francis Group

studies, patients treated with monthly injections had better visual acuity gains compared with those receiving injections as needed (pro re nata [PRN]). This has led to an enormous surge in clinic volume because patients require frequent follow-up. More recently, the VIEW (VEGF Trap-Eye: Investigation of Efficacy and Safety in Wet AMD) studies demonstrated the equivalence of aflibercept, which is administered every other month with ranibizumab administered monthly, providing the potential for less frequent dosing with a fixed treatment regimen in many patients.[7]

The treatment burden of frequent anti-VEGF injections has led several companies to pursue longer-acting anti-VEGF agents. Allergan, Inc, together with Molecular Partners, has been developing a designed ankyrin repeat protein (DARPin) that selectively binds all VEGF-A isoforms with high affinity. This genetically engineered molecule has been shown to have activity up to 3 months after injection.[8] Allergan, Inc recently announced that phase II results (unpublished at the time of publication of this book) did not warrant directly proceeding to a pivotal phase III trial, and additional phase II study is planned.[9]

Neurotech Pharmaceuticals has a proprietary Encapsulated Cell Technology (ECT) that serves as a reservoir for cells genetically modified to produce anti-VEGF antibodies. The ECT is a semipermeable capsule that allows diffusion of the anti-VEGF antibody out of and nutrients into the capsule to nourish the enclosed cells, without dispersion of the cells themselves. This implant is placed through the pars plana into the vitreous cavity and sutured to the eye wall. A low-dose phase I/II trial showed excellent safety results and a sustained effect in some patients up to 12 months.[10] A higher-dose phase I/II study is currently planned.

Another potential avenue to inhibit angiogenesis is to interrupt the translation of messenger ribonucleic acid (RNA) into VEGF or VEGF receptors. This technology—small interfering RNA (siRNA)—has generated much excitement across medicine over the past decade. Several drugs were being developed for AMD,[11] although this development has recently stalled on the first series of drugs. However, this remains a potential mechanism through which to inhibit advanced AMD.

Platelet-derived growth factor (PDGF) is another potential target because this molecule plays an important role in supporting blood vessel pericytes in choroidal neovascularization (CNV) membranes. Whereas anti-VEGF agents reduce vascular permeability and halt CNV activity, the addition of an anti-PDGF agent may stimulate regression of the CNV complex. Ophthotech Corporation is developing E10030 (Fovista), an anti-PDGF aptamer given in conjunction with ranibizumab for the treatment of wet AMD. In a phase II trial that enrolled 449 patients, the eyes that received E10030 (1.5 mg) in conjunction with ranibizumab gained 10.6 Early Treatment Diabetic Retinopathy Study (ETDRS) letters at 24 weeks, compared with 6.5 letters in the ranibizumab monotherapy arm.[12] This study differed from other recent wet AMD trials in that eligible patients had to have visual acuity of 20/63 or worse (most studies enrolled patients with vision of 20/40 or worse and even some as good as 20/25 or worse) and had to have to some component of classic CNV (most studies after the MARINA and ANCHOR trials did not differentiate between types of CNV). Despite the exclusion of a significant number of patients based on these criteria, anti-PDGF therapy, combined with an anti-VEGF agent, remains the first approach that has demonstrated efficacy better than that of anti-VEGF monotherapy. In August 2013, Ophthotech Corporation initiated a pivotal phase III trial to assess E10030 in wet AMD.

Squalamine inhibits multiple growth factors involved in angiogenesis, including VEGF, PDGF, and basic fibroblast growth factor. OHR Pharmaceutical, Inc is currently developing a topical eye drop formulation of squalamine and is currently enrolling patients in a phase II trial to assess whether a twice-daily regimen of squalamine drops can reduce or eliminate the need for intravitreal anti-VEGF injections. Prior studies evaluating the effect of intravenous squalamine on CNV showed good effect, but development was suspended because dosing required weekly infusions, and concerns were raised about the systemic side effects from intravenous administration.[13,14]

Another novel pathway under investigation for the treatment of wet AMD involves the inhibition of bioactive lipids. Bioactive lipids play an important role not only in angiogenesis but also in inflammation and fibroblast proliferation, which are important components of the neovascular process in AMD. Lpath Incorporated is currently conducting a phase II trial of iSONEP, an anti-sphingosine-1-phosphate (S1P) antibody. S1P is associated with the production and activation of VEGF, fibroblast growth factor, PDGF, interleukin-6, interleukin-8, and other growth factors implicated in the pathogenesis of wet AMD.[15] Inhibiting the action of S1P could therefore be an effective therapeutic treatment for wet AMD.

COMPLEMENT INHIBITORS

In 2005, a landmark article demonstrated a clear link between a specific complement factor H polymorphism and a genetic susceptibility to AMD.[16] Since then, research has focused on finding therapies that can disrupt the complement sequence in the hopes of inhibiting or slowing the progression from early or intermediate AMD to either advanced dry AMD (GA) or wet AMD.

Yehoshua et al[17] studied the effect of eculizumab on patients with drusen and GA. Eculizumab is a monoclonal antibody that inhibits the activation of complement factor C5, which initiates the common pathway at the end of the complement cascade. This study (the COMPLETE trial) found no difference in drusen volume, GA progression, or visual acuity in patients receiving a high dose, standard dose, or placebo after 6 months,[17] although it may not have been adequately powered to detect a meaningful difference. Interestingly, no patients treated with eculizumab converted to wet AMD during the study period, suggesting a potential role for complement inhibition in wet AMD.[18] Along these lines, Ophthotech Corporation may continue to develop ARC-1905, an aptamer that inhibits the activation of complement factor C5.

Lampalizumab is a humanized antibody fragment that inhibits complement factor D. Complement factor D is a critical component in the activation of the alternative complement pathway, which has also been implicated in the development of AMD.[19] The MAHALO (Lampalizumab [anti-factor D] in Geographic Atrophy) study was a phase II multicentered, randomized, controlled study to evaluate the safety and efficacy of lampalizumab in patients with GA.[20] This 18-month study showed that patients who were dosed monthly with an intravitreal injection of lampalizumab had a 20.4% reduction in the rate of GA progression. In a subpopulation of patients with specific exploratory biomarkers, the reduction in the rate of GA progression was 44%.[20] That study was the first to show a positive effect of complement inhibition on GA progression, and it will certainly spur additional research and development of anticomplement therapies for AMD.

However, numerous questions remain to be answered beyond the efficacy alone of such agents. Can complement inhibitors be administered locally to achieve an effect, or do they require systemic administration? Can they affect the disease when evidence of dry AMD is present, or do they need to be administered earlier in the disease process?

Finally, when used in sufficient concentrations to inhibit progression of AMD, will they also negatively affect other complement actions, such as prevention of infection?

VISUAL CYCLE MODULATORS

The complex process by which a photon of light is converted to an electric signal occurs in the photosensitive tips of the rods and cones. In this process, 11-*cis*-retinal is converted to all-*trans*-retinal, which then gets reduced and converted back to 11-*cis*-retinal in retinal pigment epithelial (RPE) cells. In addition to the desired effects, toxic by-products of the visual cycle, including A2E, are created. Accumulation of these toxic by-products has been implicated in AMD, as A2E can form free radicals, damage RPE cell membranes, inhibit RPE lysosomes, and activate the complement cascade.[21] A2E has been found to be a major component in drusen. The body's ability to remove these toxic by-products declines with age. One approach to treating AMD may be to slow the visual cycle, leading to slower accumulation of these toxic by-products.

Fenretinide was the first visual cycle modulator to be evaluated in the treatment of GA. Fenretinide binds serum retinol-binding protein (RBP) and inhibits all-*trans*-retinal transport into the retina, indirectly slowing the formation of 11-*cis*-retinal and toxic by-product production and accumulation. A multicenter, randomized, double-masked, placebo-controlled trial evaluating the effect of 100- and 300-mg daily oral doses of fenretinide did not produce a significant difference in GA lesion growth rates after 18 months.[22] Although the drug was well tolerated without significant serious adverse events, the withdrawal rates were 17.5% and 20% in the 100- and 300-mg fenretinide groups, respectively, and only 6.1% in the placebo arm. Inhibition of the visual cycle produced a delayed dark adaptation in many patients; some patients also noted dysphotopsias, both positive and negative. These side effects resolved on drug cessation.[22]

Emixustat hydrochloride is a retina-specific visual cycle modulator that inhibits RPE65, the rate-limiting enzyme in the process that converts all-*trans*-retinal back to 11-*cis*-retinal in the rod photoreceptor system. It is being investigated as a treatment for GA, and because it acts directly on RPE65, it is thought to not affect the cone photoreceptor system. Early-phase studies in healthy patients and patients with GA demonstrated a dose-dependent inhibition of the ERG, validating the proposed mode of action in this drug.[23] A phase IIb study is currently enrolling patients. The drug is being developed by Acucela, Inc.

CELL TRANSPLANTATION

Because the photoreceptors and RPE are damaged in AMD, research into replacing or supporting these cells is attractive from a scientific and clinical perspective. The use of stem cells—whether embryonic or adult—has garnered significant attention in both the scientific and popular press. The eye has been an early focus of investigation in this area because it is relatively immunoprivileged and can be easily studied and evaluated. Both regenerative and trophic stem cells are being evaluated for the treatment of advanced AMD. Regenerative cells have been differentiated into a specific cell type (eg, RPE cells) and transferred to their target tissue where they replace lost or injured cells. Trophic cells, rather than trying to replace cells, support the injured target tissue by secreting cytokines and growth factors in a paracrine fashion.

Advanced Cell Technology, Inc is currently in the midst of a phase I/II multicenter clinical trial using human embryonic stem cells that have been terminally differentiated into RPE cells. These regenerative cells are injected underneath the retina, and initial reports have not shown any specific adverse safety signals and have provided some optimism for clinical benefit.[24]

StemCells, Inc is taking a similar approach as Advanced Cell Technology, Inc, with a subretinal injection but using purified human neural stem cells (HuCNS-SC) to support photoreceptors in a trophic manner to delay or prevent subsequent atrophy. The company is currently enrolling patients in a phase I/II clinical trial to evaluate the safety of these cells in a dose-escalation study for patients with advanced dry AMD. Preclinical evaluation of these cells in a well-established rat model of photoreceptor loss showed that animals transplanted with HuCNS-SC cells had significantly less photoreceptor degeneration than control animals and sustained visual sensation during the study period.[25]

Whether stem cells will work in AMD is yet to be determined, and determining the correct way to deliver them is still another unknown variable. Both Advanced Cell Technology, Inc and StemCells, Inc are delivering their stem cells to the subretinal space by vitrectomy and transretinal delivery. In contrast, Janssen Biotech, Inc is delivering its stem cell product, derived from human umbilical tissue, to the subretinal space via a transchoroidal approach.[26] A microcatheter is inserted through a sclerotomy and choroidal incision, and viscoelastic is used to create a subretinal bleb, allowing for subretinal cannulation of the probe, which is then threaded to the temporal macula. Janssen Biotech, Inc's human umbilical tissue–derived cells act in a trophic manner to change the microenvironment and prevent (or slow) photoreceptor loss.

Neurotech Pharmaceuticals has genetically modified RPE cells to secrete ciliary neurotrophic factor (CNTF), a growth factor thought to support and enhance neural cell survival, including photoreceptors. They have placed these CNTF-secreting cells inside their proprietary Encapsulated Cell Technology (ECT). In an early clinical trial of patients with GA due to dry AMD, patients treated with this implant showed no significant adverse events, but ongoing research is still needed to fully elucidate the clinical effect.[27]

GENE THERAPY

Another exciting avenue of research for new therapeutics in AMD is gene therapy, whereby a specific gene is introduced into a diseased host cell to compensate for a missing or defective gene or where a healthy host cell is transfected and then uses its own machinery to produce a therapeutic molecule to benefit other diseased cells. The genes are delivered via viral vectors, which transfect the host cell and deliver the specific genetic material. As with stem cell therapies, the eye is an attractive organ in which to test gene therapies because of its relative immunoprivilege and the ease with which disease can be monitored. Gene therapy offers the promise of a prolonged or permanent fix, as a one-time genetic treatment can theoretically provide a lifetime of therapy.

In wet AMD, most gene therapies being studied have targeted VEGF or the VEGF receptor because this biological pathway has already demonstrated efficacy in wet AMD. Genzyme Corporation is conducting a phase I/II clinical trial of gene therapy using the adeno-associated virus 2 (AAV2) vector to deliver a gene that produces the secreted extracellular domain of VEGF receptor-1 (sFlt-1), a potent inhibitor of VEGF. Avalanche Biotechnologies is also developing an sFlt-based gene therapy loaded into an AAV vector.

Whereas Genzyme's gene is delivered via intravitreal injection, Avalanche's approach requires vitrectomy and subretinal injection.

In dry AMD, gene therapy has not been as well studied. Preclinical research continues in this important area. Hemera Biosciences, Inc is developing a complement inhibitor-based gene therapy, whereas RetroSense Therapeutics uses a photosensitivity gene—channelrhodopsin-2—to create new photosensors in the retinal cells. Animal studies using this approach have shown this treatment to be well tolerated and able to restore light perception and vision in mice and primates with naturally occurring or induced blindness from photoreceptor loss.[28,29]

SUMMARY

Advances in the management of wet AMD over the past decade have been nothing short of remarkable. Our ability to treat this once devastating disease in a manner that allows for stabilization in the majority of patients and for significant visual recovery in roughly one-third of patients has revolutionized the outlook for patients with wet AMD. New approaches to wet AMD will hopefully continue to improve outcomes and reduce the frequent need for treatment in these patients. Conversely, in dry AMD, little headway has been made in the management of this far more common condition. However, research continues, and promising trials are either ongoing or in design. We can only hope that the next decade brings equally dramatic advances in the management of both wet and dry AMD as the past decade has done for wet AMD.

REFERENCES

1. Muñoz B, West SK, Rubin GS, et al. Causes of blindness and visual impairment in a population of older Americans: the Salisbury Eye Evaluation Study. *Arch Ophthalmol*. 2000;118(6):819-825.
2. Klaver CC, Wolfs RC, Vingerling JR, et al. Age-specific prevalence and causes of blindness and visual impairment in an older population: the Rotterdam Study. *Arch Ophthalmol*. 1998;116(5):653-658.
3. Friedman DS, O'Colmain BJ, Muñoz B, et al. Prevalence of age-related macular degeneration in the United States. *Arch Ophthalmol*. 2004;122:564-572.
4. Brown DM, Kaiser PK, Michels M, et al. Ranibizumab versus verteporfin for neovascular age-related macular degeneration. *N Engl J Med*. 2006;355:1432-1444.
5. Rosenfeld PJ, Brown DM, Heier JS, et al. Ranibizumab for neovascular age-related macular degeneration. *N Engl J Med*. 2006;355:1419-1431.
6. CATT Research Group, Martin DF, Maguire MG, et al. Ranibizumab and bevacizumab for neovascular age-related macular degeneration. *N Engl J Med*. 2011;364(20):1897-1908.
7. Heier JS, Brown DM, Chong V, et al. Intravitreal aflibercept (VEGF trap-eye) in wet age-related macular degeneration. *Ophthalmology*. 2012;119(12):2537-2548.
8. Campochiaro PA, Channa R, Berger BB, et al. Treatment of diabetic macular edema with a designed ankyrin repeat protein that binds vascular endothelial growth factor: a phase I/II study. *Am J Ophthalmol*. 2013;155:697-704.
9. Cortez MF. Allergan shares fall after CEO says two studies delayed. Bloomberg.com. http://www.bloomberg.com/news/2013-05-01/allergan-shares-fall-after-ceo-says-drug-trial-will-be-delayed.html. Accessed September 6, 2013.
10. NT-503 VEGF-antagonist. Neurotech website. http://www.neurotechusa.com/VEGF-Antagonist.html. Accessed September 6, 2013.
11. Tolentino M. Interference RNA technology in the treatment of CNV. *Ophthalmol Clin North Am*. 2006;19:393-399.

12. Ophthotech's novel Anti-PDGF combination agent fovista demonstrated superior efficacy over lucentis monotherapy in large controlled wet AMD trial [press release]. New York, NY: Ophthotech Corporation; June 13, 2012.

13. Kaiser PK. Review Verteporfin photodynamic therapy and anti-angiogenic drugs: potential for combination therapy in exudative age-related macular degeneration. *Curr Med Res Opin.* 2007;23:477-487.

14. Connolly B, Desai A, Garcia CA, et al. Squalamine lactate for exudative age-related macular degeneration. *Ophthalmol Clin North Am.* 2006;19:381-391.

15. Sabbadini RA. Review targeting sphingosine-1-phosphate for cancer therapy. *Br J Cancer.* 2006; 95(9):1131-1135.

16. Edwards AO, Ritter R III, Abel KJ , et al. Complement factor H polymorphism and age-related macular degeneration. *Science.* 2005;308(5720):421-424.

17. Yehoshua Z, de Amorim Garcia Filho CA, Nunes RP, et al. Systemic complement inhibition with eculizumab for geographic atrophy in age-related macular degeneration: the COMPLETE study. *Ophthalmology.* 2014;121(3):693-701.

18. Duker JS. The COMPLETE trial for dry AMD: a look at the first phase II trial of systemic complement inhibition for dry age-related macular degeneration. *Review of Ophthalmology.* 2013;13(36). http://www.revophth.com/content/d/retina/c/36413/. Accessed September 11, 2013.

19. Loyet KM, Deforge LE, Katschke KJ Jr, et al. Activation of the alternative complement pathway in vitreous is controlled by genetics in age-related macular degeneration. *Invest Ophthalmol Vis Sci.* 2012;53(10):6628-6637.

20. Roche's lampalizumab phase II data shows benefit in patients with the advanced form of dry age-related macular degeneration. Roche website. http://www.roche.com/investors/ir_update/inv-update-2013-08-27.htm. Accessed September 6, 2013.

21. Mata NL, Kubota R, Dugal PU. Visual cycle modulation: a novel therapeutic approach for treatment of GA in dry AMD. *Retinal Physician.* 2013;10(May 1):20-23. http://www.retinalphysician.com/articleviewer.aspx?articleID=108371. Accessed September 6, 2013.

22. Mata NL, Lichter JB, Vogel R, et al. Investigation of oral fenretinide for treatment of geographic atrophy in age-related macular degeneration. *Retina.* 2013;33(3):498-507.

23. Kubota R1, Boman NL, David R, et al. Safety and effect on rod function of ACU-4429, a novel small-molecule visual cycle modulator. *Retina.* 2012;32(1):183-188.

24. Schwartz SD, Hubschman JP, Heilwell G, et al. Embryonic stem cell trials for macular degeneration: a preliminary report. *Lancet.* 2012;379:713-720.

25. McGill TJ, Cottam B, Lu B, et al. Transplantation of human central nervous system stem cells—neuroprotection in retinal degeneration. *Eur J Neurosci.* 2012;35:468-477.

26. Ho AC. Human adult umbilical stem cells potential treatment for atrophic AMD: a phase 1 clinical trial is assessing safety. *Retina Today.* 2011;October:59-61.

27. Jaffe GJ, Tao W. A phase 2 study of encapsulated CNTF-secreting cell implant (NT-501) in patients with geographic atrophy associated with dry AMD—18-month results. Paper presented at: American Society of Retina Specialists 28th Annual Meeting; August 28-September 1, 2010; Vancouver, Canada.

28. Ivanova E, Hwang GS, Pan ZH, Troilo D. Evaluation of AAV-mediated expression of Chop2-GFP in the marmoset retina. Paper presented at: Association for Research in Vision and Ophthalmology (ARVO) Annual Meeting; May 2010; Orlando, FL.

29. Bi A, Cui J, Ma YP, et al. Ectopic expression of a microbial-type rhodopsin restores visual responses in mice with photoreceptor degeneration. *Neuron.* 2006;50(1):23-33.

Appendix

ABBREVIATIONS

AMD: age-related macular degeneration

ANCHOR: Anti-VEGF Antibody for the Treatment of Predominantly Classic Choroidal Neovascularisation in AMD

AREDS: Age-Related Eye Disease Study

BCVA: best corrected visual acuity

BLamD: basal laminar deposits

BLinD: basal linear deposits

CNV: choroidal neovascularization

CSC: central serous chorioretinopathy

ECM: extracellular matrix

EOG: electro-oculogram

ERG: electroretinogram

FA: fluorescein angiography

FAF: fundus autofluroscence

FAZ: foveal avascular zone

GA: geographic atrophy

hyperAF: hyperautofluorescent

hypoAF: hypoautofluorescent

ICGA: indocyanine green angiography

IOP: intraocular pressure

MacTel: macular telangiectasia

MARINA: Minimally Classic/Occult Trial of the Anti-VEGF Antibody Ranibizumab in the Treatment of Neovascular AMD

MPS: Macular Photocoagulation Study

OCT: optical coherence tomography

Duker JS, Witkin AJ, eds.
*Age-Related Macular Degeneration:
Current Management (pp. 147-148)*
© 2015 Taylor & Francis Group

PCV: polypoidal choroidal vasculopathy

PPV: pars plana vitrectomy

PRN: pro re nata

RAP: retinal angiomatous proliferation

RPE: retinal pigment epithelium

RPED: retinal pigment epithelial detachment

TAP: Treatment of AMD With Photodynamic Therapy study

tPA: tissue plasminogen activator

VEGF: vascular endothelial growth factor

VIP: Verteporfin in Photodynamic Therapy study

FINANCIAL DISCLOSURES

Dr. Anita Agarwal has no financial or proprietary interest in the materials presented herein.

Dr. Sophie J. Bakri has no financial or proprietary interest in the materials presented herein.

Dr. Christopher J. Brady has no financial or proprietary interest in the materials presented herein.

Dr. Jay S. Duker has no financial or proprietary interest in the materials presented herein.

Dr. Sunir J. Garg has disclosed financial relationships with Allergan, Genentech, and Regeneron.

Dr. Roger A. Goldberg has no financial or proprietary interest in the materials presented herein.

Dr. Jeffrey S. Heier is a scientific advisor to Acucela, Alcon, Allergan, Bayer, Genentech, Genzyme/Sanofi, Merz, Neurotech, Notal Vision, Ohr Pharmaceuticals, Oraya, and Regeneron and has received research funds from Acucela, Alcon, Genentech, Genzyme, Lpath, Notal Vision, Novartis, Ohr Pharmaceutical, Ophthotech, QLT, and Regeneron.

Dr. S.K. Steven Houston III has no financial or proprietary interest in the materials presented herein.

Dr. Kapil G. Kapoor has no financial or proprietary interest in the materials presented herein.

Dr. Nora M.V. Laver has no financial or proprietary interest in the materials presented herein.

Dr. Sana Nadeem has no financial or proprietary interest in the materials presented herein.

Dr. Llewelyn J. Rao has no financial or proprietary interest in the materials presented herein.

Dr. Carl D. Regillo has no financial or proprietary interest in the materials presented herein.

Dr. Elias Reichel has no financial or proprietary interest in the materials presented herein.

Dr. Philip J. Rosenfeld has no financial or proprietary interest in the materials presented herein.

Dr. Chirag P. Shah has been a subinvestigator on studies with the following sponsors: Alcon, Alimera, Allergan, Fovea, Genentech, Genzyme, Partners, Neovista, Novartis, Ophthotech, and Regeneron.

Dr. Lawrence J. Singerman has no financial or proprietary interest in the materials presented herein.

Dr. Mariana R. Thorell has no financial or proprietary interest in the materials presented herein.

Dr. Michael D. Tibbetts has no financial or proprietary interest in the materials presented herein.

Dr. Nadia K. Waheed has no financial or proprietary interest in the materials presented herein.

Dr. Andre J. Witkin has no financial or proprietary interest in the materials presented herein.

INDEX